Praise for EATING LESS:

'Gillian Riley's approach is clear, simple and powerful in its effect on people's lives. For smoking and overeating, her work is excellent in both areas. Simply the best.'
LESLIE KENTON, HEALTH EXPERT AND WRITER

'Immensely interesting and helpful. Empowers those who previously have felt themselves to be the victims of dieting and dietary advice.'
DOROTHY ROWE, PSYCHOLOGIST AND WRITER

'The utter simplicity of its message and techniques makes *Eating Less* easy to start and continue with a programme that revolutionises your attitude to eating and weight.'
SARAH LITVINOFF

'Whereas most diet books have you focus on the latest fad and fashion in dieting, this book has you focus on YOU. Make a covenant with yourself — Eat Less! This is Gillian Riley's simple message. Through Gillian's no-nonsense approach to the nature of desire and addiction, you will gain wisdom about how you can make such a covenant your living reality.'
MITRA RAY, PHD, CELL BIOLOGIST AND WRITER

'One woman I worked with recently had undergone therapy at a NHS funded clinic and she said your book gave her more insight in the few days she took to read it than months of counselling.'
MAGGIE PRESTON, MA, COUNSELLOR

EATING LESS

Say goodbye to overeating

GILLAN RILEY

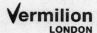

Vermilion
LONDON

First published in the UK in 1998 by Vermilion, an imprint of Ebury Publishing
This revised and updated edition published by Vermilion in 2005

Ebury Publishing is a Random House Group company

The Random House Group Limited Reg. No. 954009

Addresses for companies within the Random House Group can be found at
www.randomhouse.co.uk

A CIP catalogue record for this book is available from the British Library

ISBN 978 0 09 190247 6

Copies are available at special rates for bulk orders.
Contact the sales development team on 020 7840 8487 or visit
www.booksforpromotions.co.uk for more information.

To buy books by your favourite authors and register for offers, visit
www.randomhouse.co.uk

The Random House Group Limited supports The Forest Stewardship Council (FSC®), the leading international forest certification organisation. Our books carrying the FSC label are printed on FSC® certified paper. FSC is the only forest certification scheme endorsed by the leading environmental organisations, including Greenpeace. Our paper procurement policy can be found at
www.randomhouse.co.uk/environment

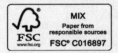

Printed and bound in Great Britain by Clays Ltd, St Ives PLC

Although every effort has been made to ensure that the contents of this book are accurate, it must not be treated as a substitute for qualified medical advice. Neither the Author nor the Publisher can be held responsible for any loss or claim arising out of the use, or misuse, of the suggestions made or the failure to take medical advice.

Contents

Acknowledgements

I am grateful to everyone who gave their permission to quote from research papers and books, especially Drs Nathaniel Branden and Jeffrey M. Schwartz. I have made all reasonable efforts to contact copyright holders for permission, and apologise for any omissions or errors in the form of credit given. Corrections can be made in future printings.

My thanks also go to my clients and readers who wrote their stories for this edition.

Introduction

When it comes to making changes in your eating – whether you think of it as dieting, losing weight or healthy eating – certain approaches are usually suggested. This book will have you question them.

- *MYTH: Wait until you're hungry before you eat.* Using hunger as your guide can be inconvenient, impractical and very difficult to interpret accurately. Much research has shown that hunger is unreliable as a signal to eat.
- *MYTH: Stop eating when you're full.* Most people don't feel the 'fullness' of what they ate until quite a few minutes *after* finishing their meal. If you tend to overeat, this is too late.
- *MYTH: Sugar is addictive, so the only solution is to abstain.* It's a very tall order never to eat sugar again. If your success depends on abstinence it will be fragile, and once broken there's no other strategy to use.
- *MYTH: Stop eating sugar, wheat and/or processed food, and your cravings will disappear.* There are plenty of yo-yo dieters who have kept to healthy regimes for months at a time but returned to overeating because their desire for these foods resurfaced.

- *MYTH: Eat anything you fancy and trust your body to tell you what it needs.* If this worked, there would be none of the many ailments and diseases associated with poor nutrition. This book shows you how to overcome your attraction to the manufactured 'non-foods' that can make you ill.
- *MYTH: Avoid temptations and keep yourself busy to stop thinking about food.* As you may already know, this strategy will only take you so far. As with any problem in life, evading it doesn't resolve it in the long term.
- *MYTH: Don't eat while watching television.* This advice is to keep your attention on your food, but nobody suggests you shouldn't have a conversation at a meal! You can eat less at meals – and talk, read a newspaper or watch a programme at the same time, if that's what you want to do.
- *MYTH: Overeating is the result of unresolved emotional issues.* Yet many people overeat when they're happy and enjoying themselves. It can be liberating to discover a way to overcome overeating without delving into your past.

Welcome to a completely different solution.

CHAPTER 1

Food Addiction

I have just given up spinach for Lent.
F. SCOTT FITZGERALD

Are you addicted to food? If you struggle with your answer, please know that addiction isn't necessarily extreme. A two-a-day smoker can be described as addicted. It would be fair to say that they are less addicted than a chain-smoker would be, but the same process is involved.

Food addiction comes in a vast array of shapes and sizes. It can apply to those of normal weight as well as to the overweight and obese. It can even apply to those who are underweight, because some people can stay very slim on nothing but highly addictive junk food.

This book explains how to overcome food addiction, large and small. One problem we face is that food addiction is such a pervasive and established part of our culture, it can be hard even to see it in the first place. See if any of these characteristics come close to describing the way you are with food:

▌ you know you eat way too much at mealtimes but don't feel satisfied with smaller portions

- you continue to snack after an evening meal
- you open a packet of biscuits intending to eat one or two but rarely leave anything but crumbs
- you think about food too much of the time
- you feel hungry much of the time
- you feel hungry after eating a substantial meal
- you often feel uncomfortable or even unwell after eating (sleepy, bloated or nauseous, for example)
- you rarely, if ever, feel a genuine, natural hunger
- you are fearful of feeling genuine hunger
- you eat much too quickly and find it tough to slow down
- you go into a kind of trance sometimes and don't even know you are eating
- you rarely eat the recommended 'five-a-day' of fruit and vegetables
- you find it very challenging to stick to a diet, or, when you do, you regain any weight lost
- from time to time you feel compelled to binge on unhealthy food you don't usually eat, only to feel regretful and upset about it later
- you are not in the best possible health, perhaps suffering from heartburn, constipation or fatigue
- you rely for energy on stimulants such as sugar, caffeine and/or nicotine
- you care a great deal more about your family's healthy eating than your own
- you regularly feel guilty or regretful about what or how much you eat
- you consistently make and break promises to yourself about what you are and are not going to eat
- you know you eat too much unhealthy food but dislike eating vegetables, whole grains and/or fruit

■ your life, and especially your mood, is ruled by the
scales

It may well be that practically everybody experiences some
of these from time to time, but remember that addiction is a
matter of degree. There's no clear-cut line that defines an
addictive relationship with food *precisely* – and there never
will be. This doesn't mean that food addiction doesn't exist,
and if you experience any of the above as ongoing *problems*
in your life, it can actually be helpful to understand that in
terms of addiction.

Not everyone agrees that food is addictive. My con-
viction has come from my experience of helping people to
stop smoking. Smokers frequently smoke instead of eat,
and, especially when stopping smoking, eat instead of
smoke. Tobacco is widely accepted as being addictive, and
for many people the desire to smoke and the desire to eat
become interchangeable – and at times *indistinguishable*.

There are even some smokers who aren't particularly
addicted to nicotine, but far more addicted to food. These
smokers can take or leave cigarettes, and the only reason
they smoke is in order to control their eating and weight.
They are not really smokers; they are overeaters who smoke.
The smoking part of stopping smoking is relatively easy for
them. Their challenge is in facing up to their eating
addiction without cigarettes.

Another similarity between smoking and overeating is
their almost identical – and rather dismal – rates of relapse.
One characteristic that defines addiction is repeated failure
to gain control, and it is well known that both smokers and
dieters have great difficulty in maintaining their good
intentions in the longer term. Studies report that out of

every 100 smokers making a serious attempt to quit, as many as 95 of them will return to smoking within a year. The same failure rate is often quoted with regard to dieting, and one survey reported results that were even worse. An astounding 99 per cent either didn't lose the weight they had wanted to lose or regained the weight within a year, according to this study, conducted in England in 2003. (1)

In recent years, scientists have begun to uncover bio-chemical reactions to food that are consistent with addiction. It seems that fats and simple sugars in particular act in the brain in very similar ways to nicotine and other addictive drugs. (2)

By saying food is addictive we don't create a problem but face an existing one with the truth. Far from being a judgement – another stick to beat yourself with about what you eat – we can use the concept of addiction as the explanation for overeating. The point is that it's only when you understand addiction and how it works that you can appreciate the strategies needed to tackle it.

Even so, calling overeating an addiction raises many more questions than it answers. Each different addiction – whether it's nicotine, caffeine or whatever – has its own particular characteristics. Being a smoker is clearly not the same as being addicted to crack cocaine. Heroin addiction is not the same as compulsive gambling. What's important, though, are the characteristics they share that cause them to be called addictions. Let's see what those characteristics are and how they relate to food.

Aspects of Addiction

Addictive Desire – 'I want it.'

Perhaps the most obvious characteristic of addiction is a concept so familiar we have many words to describe it: desire, craving, impulse, compulsion, urge, yearning, longing, anticipation and even obsession. When you are addicted to something you are attracted to it, and it is this attraction that makes it tough to control.

This is implicit in the concept of addiction: it's something you have difficulty *not* doing because at the same time as wanting to stop doing it, you also want to do it! This is why, over and over again, you overeat, only to regret it later, and find it so very difficult to change those patterns in a way that lasts.

It's often claimed that this excessive, addictive appetite is caused by the sudden fall of blood glucose levels caused by eating certain kinds of carbohydrates. We'll take a look at this in Chapter 8, but it's only one part of the whole story.

To a very large extent, addictive desire is the product of a special kind of memory. It's known as a *conditioned response*, which refers to the automatic associations the brain makes with certain cues. For example, if I snack in front of the television every evening, then I have conditioned myself to expect a snack whenever I sit down to watch television. My brain produces the conditioned response – the addictive desire – whether or not I'm naturally hungry and no matter what's happening with my blood glucose. This conditioning is a key factor in all addictions, but it's especially important in dealing with smoking and eating because the cues are such an unavoidable part of our daily lives.

The addictive desire to eat can masquerade as hunger, both before and after eating. This is one reason why the advice to 'eat when you're hungry and stop when you're full' is too simplistic. Hunger and fullness are very much influenced by our addiction, as we'll see in Chapter 8.

Everything in this book is aimed at showing you what to do about this addictive desire as it's the core issue in dealing with addictive behaviour.

Interaction of Body and Mind – 'I need it.'

When you call something an addiction (rather than just a bad habit) you are saying that there's a certain kind of body chemistry involved. Biochemically speaking, an addiction takes its grip on us through our natural reward system. (3)

This system motivates us to seek out positive, life-enhancing rewards, by releasing chemicals in our brains (the most significant are thought to be dopamine, serotonin and beta-endorphins), which reinforce any beneficial behaviour. Eating *any* food is beneficial behaviour, of course, but this response seems to be exaggerated with certain kinds of food.

Our brains get the message that fats and simple sugars in particular are more rewarding than raw vegetables! For most overeaters, the conditioned response – the feeling of addictive desire – tends to be stronger for the more addictive kinds of food. And the more we eat them the more we reinforce our attraction towards them.

Fortunately for us, we have minds as well as brains. The good news is that the right sort of mental attention you bring to this can and does have an effect on the working of the brain. Neuroscientist Jeffrey Schwartz writes, 'The seemingly simple act of "paying attention" produces real and powerful physical changes in the brain.' (4)

This is crucial to our recovery, as we'll discover later on – and it is something that has been largely overlooked in this field. Approaches to food addiction usually take the line that since biochemistry is involved, the solution must either be pharmacological (an antidepressant or an appetite suppressant) or abstinence (from sugar or from all carbo-hydrates, for example).

None of these solutions recognises the considerable power of the mind. After all, it's impossible not to have any attitude at all with regard to food, so your mind is involved whether you want to acknowledge it or not. This means that purely physical solutions are only going to work up to a point, if at all. Of course, biochemistry is involved, but it's your *attitude* that makes the crucial difference, and with the right attitude it's entirely possible to think your way through this and out the other side. The book that explains how to do this is in your hands right now.

Downside – 'It's bad for me.'

When we call something an addiction we imply that there's a problem; some kind of damage to health, wealth and self-esteem. We may be addicted to things that are good for us, such as food or exercise, but the part we call 'addiction' is, by definition, the part that is harming us in some way.

Addictions never contribute to our wellbeing. Something that is essential such as sleeping, although repeated daily all through our lives and something we feel compelled to do at times, isn't called an addiction. We genuinely need to sleep for at least a few out of every 24 hours, so there's no problem. In fact, we have problems if we *don't* do it!

Sooner or later the downside becomes too much of a problem, and when the addiction continues despite the downside, guilt becomes an added problem. The most obvious downside to addictive overeating is excess weight. But, as you will see in the next three chapters, it will serve you to become aware of all the other things you inevitably sacrifice in the pursuit of your particular 'fix'.

As well as being the unwelcome consequences, the downside adds power to an addiction, making it even more compelling. For example, the fact that smoking is regarded as forbidden makes it more exciting for some people than it would otherwise be, especially the young. Food addiction may seem innocent but the same mechanism is at work. 'Banned' foods become naughty fun and can even create a very difficult state of obsession. Many people overeat as a rebellion against the pressure to diet, to lose weight or just to eat any less at all.

Chapter 5 is all about understanding this rebellious reaction to the idea of restricting or depriving yourself, and how to eliminate it entirely.

Pleasure and Satisfaction – 'It's my treat.'

We find it pleasurable to satisfy our addictive desire – and, of course, pleasure is very much a matter of personal preference. Personally, I can't think of much that's less pleasurable than gambling – but there may well be compulsive gamblers who are indifferent to chocolate-covered raisins.

Addiction lives in the world of sensation, supported by placing the highest value on the pursuit of immediate pleasure. It's fuelled by a sense of excitement, satisfaction or reward. This is why we have the addictive desire; we want to repeat the things we enjoy. There can come a time when you get little or no pleasure from an addiction, often because the downside has become too overwhelming and even frightening. But at some time in the development of the addiction, some amount of pleasure was involved.

When it comes to dealing with food addiction, one difficulty is that pleasure and satisfaction are perfectly normal, appropriate and even necessary responses to eating food. This gives credibility to the familiar justification for overeating: 'I enjoy my food – what's wrong with that?'

Many people overeat as a rebellion against the pressure to diet, to lose weight or just to eat any less at all.

Maybe one way to think about it is that you are getting *too much* pleasure from eating, and nothing will change for you unless you forgo some of that pleasure. That may initially seem impossible – even unthinkable – but this is where we're headed: to eat less and to feel so good about it that you want to continue, even though there is temptation sometimes. The challenge first of all is to recognise the difference between a more appropriate level of enjoyment and the satisfaction of addictive desire, and you will be learning exactly how to do that.

Altered State of Consciousness – 'It cheers me up.'

To varying degrees, addictions temporarily change the way we think and feel; they make us high, drugged, 'absent-minded' or numbed in some way. Overeaters can go into a kind of daze even while eating a perfectly ordinary meal. A food binge can create a state of intoxication or stupor not unlike that produced by alcohol.

This altered state of consciousness can create a buffer between us and our feelings which brings us a sense of comfort, and this is why we often turn to our addictions when we are unhappy or stressed. A number of books focus on this exclusively as the cause of overeating – but do keep in mind that a great many people also eat addictively when they are happy and content. A perfectly happy family can have an addictive relationship with food as much as one that's perfectly dysfunctional!

Satisfying our addictive desire usually brings us a sense of pleasure, so there aren't many circumstances in which we won't want to do that. When you learn about addiction and the addictive appetite you'll be able to see your way through this. You'll be able to experience for yourself that the 'comfort' you get from overeating may not be so much of a benefit as it sometimes seems.

Withdrawal Symptoms – 'It's awful when I stop.'

Withdrawal is the term given to anything unpleasant or challenging that happens when you stop an addictive behaviour. There are a number of different aspects to withdrawal.

You could get physical symptoms of detoxification such as headaches, fatigue or aches and pains, but only if you make quite a dramatic change from a very unhealthy to a healthy eating style. This comes from the rapid release of toxins, and although it can feel like illness, it's really just your body recovering from the abuse of the addictive food. These symptoms are temporary and not really too troublesome. Also, they're not an essential part of the process; if you want to make changes more gradually, that's fine.

Consider, though, that this aspect of withdrawal could be part of your life already. A whole range of ailments could be reactions to whatever addictive junk food you consumed the previous day. You might regard your lack of energy, low mood and inability to concentrate as permanent and inevitable features in your life, and only see their connection with food when you start to eat in a healthier way.

Sugar in particular is well known for its addictive properties. One study of rats hooked on sugar received some attention in the newspapers. The detail that sparked interest was that the rats' teeth were chattering uncontrollably during withdrawal. Eating any food, and sugar in particular, increases the release of beta-endorphins (endogenous opioids, which are completely natural) so it's likely that some drug-like withdrawal could occur. However, the rats consumed massive amounts of sugar and were put into withdrawal in an extreme and artificial way. Sugar certainly is addictive and presents us with a challenge but your symptoms won't be so alarming.

Far more important is the psychological side of withdrawal, the changes you will be making in the ways you think. It's very common for people to try to take control of an addiction without considering the psychological side of withdrawal, and this is exactly why they fail in the longer term. Taking control of overeating, as any other addiction, is a major change, and nobody does something like that without some kind of inner struggle, a process of re-evaluation. *Psychological withdrawal is the difficulty in making a real change – and it's an essential part of the process.* This book shows you how, but you are the only one who's ever going to be able to put it into practice.

Secondary Conditioning – 'I love everything about it.'

We get pleasure not only from an addiction, but also from all kinds of things directly associated with it. Heroin addicts can get as much excitement from procuring their drug and preparing it for use as in doing it. Smokers often develop a fondness for their lighters and the packet design of their brand of cigarettes. Some alcoholics thoroughly enjoy their active social life only because it's integral to their drinking; without the booze the friends would be worthless.

In the same way, shopping for food, preparation of food and any event which includes eating can carry a special significance for the addicted eater. Food could be your hobby or even your career. Of course, the difficulty with food addiction is that it all seems so completely natural and normal. It's important, though, to see that this addiction is made up of the same things as other addictions.

Susceptibility – 'My whole family's prone to it.'

Everyone's body is different. We aren't all born with the potential to become world-class athletes, opera singers – or alcoholics. We can only work with what we're given. What we may have been given is a predisposition to become addicted to things in general, and to food in particular.

It's estimated that about one quarter of the general population produces far too much insulin and glucose in response to carbohydrates. These are likely to be the people most susceptible to food addiction and to gaining body fat more easily. Another quarter of the population is thought to be unaffected by carbohydrate intake, no matter how much they consume. The remaining 50 per cent lie in between, with an increasing tendency to develop problems with insulin and glucose if they aren't careful about their carbohydrate consumption.

Some studies indicate that an addiction to sugar in particular may be somehow similar to alcoholism, and that those with a family history of alcoholism may be more susceptible to food addiction. (5)

These could be purely physical, genetic factors in addictive eating, but remember, it's just one part of the whole picture. It may well go some way in explaining why one person or family overeats when another doesn't, but it doesn't mean you won't be able to make real, lasting changes for yourself.

Exposure – 'Everyone's doing it.'

Before we can take up a particular addiction, we must have access to it, and the more widespread it is in our community, the more likely we are to get involved. If all my friends smoke, I am much more likely to join in, especially if I'm young.

Of course, most of us have access to too much food, and especially too much addictive food, but some social groups encourage its consumption. You may be part of a family or group of friends that regards addictive overeating as normal, perhaps even beneficial, such as when people say 'I've got a healthy appetite'.

Our culture encourages addictive eating. The food industry is chiefly concerned with selling its products, which means promoting the more popular, addictive foods – mostly processed products which contain the bad fats, sugar, wheat, potatoes and salt – rather than health. 'Health' is a good marketing strategy, but is rarely, if ever, much more than that.

Advertising and availability make addictive food seem a normal and natural part of everyday life. As a result, a great many of us have become confused about food, unable to appreciate or even care about the essential difference between a bag of crisps and an apple, for example. (6)

When an addictive behaviour is so accepted within a culture, it can make it almost impossible to see addiction at work behind it. For example, in many parts of the world so many people smoke, it's considered odd if you don't. This doesn't mean the smokers are not addicted; it just means that that particular society has a different attitude towards that addiction. That was the situation in the UK in the 1940s, 50s and even into the 60s. Doctors would recommend taking up smoking to stressed or anxious patients, and endorse particular brands in advertisements. A carton of cigarettes was an appropriate and acceptable gift in any social circle. These days, your social circle might feel the same way about a box of chocolates. Maybe it's time to think again about this kind of convention. (7)

Your social group may consider it normal to eat a portion of chips every day for lunch. Your family may think it perfectly normal to eat white bread. I was raised in such a family. My point is that just because everybody around you does it, this doesn't mean it isn't addictive eating.

Living in a food-addicted culture doesn't mean you can't do anything about your own eating. The techniques you'll learn in this book will enable you to assert yourself, to say 'no thanks' when it's appropriate instead of always going along with everyone else.

Tolerance – 'I've got a big appetite and a sweet tooth.'

If you've been eating in addictive ways for years, your body has adapted itself by developing some degree of tolerance.

> *When an addictive behaviour is so accepted within a culture, it can make it almost impossible to see addiction at work behind it.*

Our bodies always try to adapt to and endure the abuse we inflict on them. For example, we could take small amounts of poison, gradually increase the dose and eventually survive what would otherwise, on the first try, be fatal. Tolerance means we get accustomed to unnatural substances, which is why doses often increase.

People may start smoking only one or two cigarettes a day, but over time increase to 20 or 30 a day. The body becomes tolerant of nicotine and more is required in order to achieve the same effect. If a non-smoker tried to smoke 30 in one day, they would feel absolutely dreadful because they haven't built up the tolerance.

With food addiction, our stomachs expand so we can tolerate – and therefore come to expect – larger amounts. We also develop tolerance for the quality of our food, which means that the more addictive food you eat, the more addictive food you'll want to eat. You might call it a sweet tooth, but it's really an addiction to sugar.

People often say their taste buds change after making changes in what they eat. Larger amounts of sugar and fat, for example, don't appeal as much as they once did because the tolerance for them has faded. This is good news, because you can begin to see that it isn't 'you' who has to consume all that chocolate cake or whatever, but a conditioned version of you who has built up a degree of tolerance over the years. That means you really can change, and as you do, different kinds and amounts of food will start to appeal to you and satisfy you more.

Justification – 'Life's too short' and Denial – 'It's not going to kill me.'

All addictions are supported by ways of thinking that become so familiar it can be tough to separate the truth from the illusion. These beliefs work hand in hand to encourage you to satisfy your addictive appetite. For example, you might justify overeating by telling yourself you deserve it. Your denial could be that you are eating far too much, or that it's bad for you in any way.

Justification and denial are such a powerful part of addiction it's essential to break their hold. After all, if your life will fall apart without it and it isn't doing you any harm, why would you ever want to stop overeating?

Justification and denial help you to feel less guilty about addictive eating. Whenever the denial is challenged – when you get ill for example – and you realise the overeating is in fact damaging, the more you'll rely on your justifications, and the more convincing they need to be. This tends to create some fear at the thought of eating less, because you are so convinced that you are dependent on it in some significant way.

This doesn't mean the justifications and the fear they create are your best guides to your wisest decisions. Facing the fear is always part of the process because it's only by facing fear that you can overcome it. We'll look at justifications in more detail in Chapter 9.

As an example of denial, one client, Janet, swore to me that she couldn't think of one reason to cut back on her overeating other than to lose weight. She thought and thought, and looked at me as if I were mad to suggest such a silly idea. But only two weeks earlier, she had cancelled a session because of a migraine which she had told me was brought on by overeating the day before. Her addicted mind had, quite automatically, ignored this.

A common example of denial is found in the experience of repeatedly overeating and regretting it later on. At the point when you are buying this food in the shop, the denial means you totally forget about the regret you'll feel later. You've no recollection at all about how bad you feel after you've eaten these particular things, even though you've done it over and over again. All you remember at the time is how yummy they are. So you buy them, you eat them and *then* you remember! 'Oh no! I feel ghastly. I wish I hadn't eaten all that. Why do I always do this?'

Denial is tricky to overcome because by definition it's hidden. Take note of any physical symptoms of ill health you have, especially persistent ones. Is it possible they have anything to do with either the quality or the quantity of the food you eat? The best approach is to assume that you have some degree of denial going on. It's automatic, and in Chapter 10 we'll see why. Once you've seen it for what it is, it's difficult to go back into denial, which makes it much easier to stick to what you really want to be doing. (8)

As well as the truths you keep hidden from yourself, addiction often involves keeping things from other people as well, perhaps by overeating only when alone and hiding the wrappers. Most addicts keep crucial details of their addictions secret, and may even try to keep the whole addiction secret, especially from certain people. Of course, it's difficult to hide the effects of addictive eating, which is why so many of us become obsessed with weight loss: it's evidence that other people can see. It's easy to forget just how much you've eaten but much tougher to deny that you simply *cannot* get into your favourite pair of jeans.

Conflict of Values – 'I'm confused about it.'

Anyone addicted to anything has experienced some degree of ambivalence about it at some point, when they are not at all sure whether they want to make any changes. This is because practising an addiction means you make one value – satisfying the addiction – more important than another value, such as being in the best possible health. When you begin the process of taking control of overeating, you start to create a new priority in your values: *I* matter here, the quality of *my* life matters, *my* health matters – to *me*. This doesn't happen automatically, and it probably won't feel natural at first. You need to make deliberate choices to change things, and initially you may feel torn in two.

The process of breaking free from any addiction is the process of resolving this conflict by changing your priorities. This is crucial, because any addiction is strengthened by the confusion and inconsistency of purpose that surrounds it.

Action – 'It's what I do.'

For me, one of the most fascinating aspects of addictions is that they involve behaviour – things you do. However hard you may try, you can't get away from the fact of the actions you have or have not taken. You could affirm your commitment to your health over and over again, but if you follow that with the actions of addictive overeating, your health and self-esteem will suffer.

This can be a hard lesson to learn, but it has its bright side. Changing your actions – your behaviour, if done correctly, has tremendous psychological and spiritual rewards.

Addiction in Mind

When we think about food addiction, our first images are perhaps the most dramatic and obvious. It's a midnight binge, eating spoonfuls of creamy, sugary goo in a semi-conscious daze. It's eating when you're depressed or angry. It's eating two whole chocolate cakes for dinner. It's eating too quickly and going back for second and third helpings. But when we recognise that addiction is a matter of degree, we can begin to see the enormous range of insidious and subtle ways it influences our relationship with food.

Naming overeating as an addiction opens the door to the solutions. After all, if food is addictive, then maybe the *only* way to gain peace of mind is by facing up to that truth. If food is addictive, then telling an overeater to follow a diet or particular dietary recommendations – *any diet or recommendations* – may be just as ineffective as telling a smoker to stop smoking. The real question is, *how*? And, more importantly, how to do it in a way that lasts.

In this book we will approach taking control of over-eating from the perspective of psychological addiction: the aspect of addiction that exists in the way in which we think. We will look at three factors in particular: what they are, why they can hinder your progress, and how to change them when they do. These factors are:

1   **what motivates you:** the question of why you might want to make any changes in what and how much you eat
2   **your sense of choice:** the degree of freedom or restriction you feel when you make changes in what and how much you eat
3   **your addictive desire:** your attitude towards feeling tempted by your addictive appetite

When you start to make alterations in these three ways of thinking, your relationship with food changes as a direct result. You will eat in less addictive ways, and those changes will more easily become a normal part of your life. We will be exploring the first of these – your motivation – over the next three chapters.

IN OTHER WORDS: GILLIAN

At the end of each chapter you'll find a section like this written by someone who read the first edition of this book, and in some cases also attended one of my courses. This first one, though, is my story – because I do eat, and I certainly have the ability to overeat. Every word I write on this subject is tested by my personal experience, and there ➤

are no strategies or advice in this book that I don't follow myself. Left to my own devices, so to speak, I'd consume nothing but high-fat, sugary or salty, addictive 'food' all day, every day. I've been as big as a house in the past, and if I didn't know better I would be so again.

I used to believe that I was born fat and that's just the way I was made. I have photos of myself as an infant looking just like a Buddha. It wasn't until my 30s that I began to consider that my weight might have something to do with what I was eating.

I have broken a great many addictive patterns of eating, such as eating crisps every time I went shopping and snacking in the evenings while watching TV. Now I almost never think of eating in these situations. These habits haven't been replaced with any other behaviours or food and I've not avoided the situations at all.

I strongly suspect that I now have as happy a relationship with food as anyone you'll ever meet. My weight fluctuates very little and I am in no sense at war with myself, either with my shape or my food. I don't abstain from any particular kind of food in order to maintain control. I don't eat squid because I dislike the idea of it, but I'll eat almost anything else. My aim is to make the best choices in what I eat most days, and I don't worry at all about odd lapses when I'm socialising.

I'm not skinny and don't want to be. I'm a healthy weight and believe I'm as healthy as I can possibly be without being fanatical, anti-social or otherwise faddy and weird about it. Healthy eating has been my main objective with food for over 20 years. I have every ➤

*intention of living a long life, but more importantly to me,
a healthy one all the way into my old age.*

*I am keenly aware of my addictive thinking, and I
believe it is nothing but this awareness that gives me the
ability to stay in control of my eating. This approach, which
I'll explain to you in this book, is all I'll ever use or need.*

Taking Control

- These sections will suggest mental and written exercises,
  and new ways of thinking for you to bring into your life. They
  will enable you to integrate this approach so that you can
  make the lasting changes you want.

- You may want to read this book on your own, or create a
  group to meet and discuss it on a regular basis. Alternatively,
  you may want to find a counsellor or therapist with whom you
  can explore these themes. All of these are possibilities for
  you to choose from, depending on your needs and circumstances. It's impossible to be too specific because each of us
  will have varying degrees of difficulty with these topics.

- My main advice at the start, as I advise each of my clients, is
  that you don't make this technique the subject of general
  discussion with family and friends. Your relationship with the
  food you eat is personal, private and unique; making a change
  in that relationship needs to be personal and private too. The
  people in your life may eat with you and even cook for you, but
  ultimately it's up to you and you alone what goes in your
  mouth.

  You might be tempted to explain what you've learned in

this book in order to help others with their eating problems. *I strongly advise you against this* as it could be met with resistance and is likely to impair your own progress. By all means let them know about this book, but then leave them alone to decide whether or not they want to read and use it.

My suggestion to keep it private may seem unusual. If you often talk with friends about food and weight issues, this advice may seem difficult to follow, and at this stage in the book you may not see the point of it. However, it makes the technique much easier to use, and as you read on you will see why. I'm mentioning it at the beginning so that you can give it a lower profile right from the start.

- As you read on, it's likely you'll have some concerns about what all this will lead to in the future. What will your life be like if you get involved with this book? Will you be able to cope with parties, family gatherings and holidays? And will you continue to use these principles even though you've given up on things you've tried before? You may even find that the thought of success is just as frightening as predicting failure.

Be careful, because although worries such as these are perfectly normal and understandable, they can easily turn into the self-fulfilling prophecy: 'I'll never be able to keep this up, so I won't bother trying too hard in the first place.' Counter this thinking by bringing yourself back to the here and now. Remind yourself that the future hasn't happened yet; it exists only in your thoughts. The more you stay focused on the present time – whatever is happening *right now* – the less you'll fear change and the easier it will be for you to stay positive about the changes you want to make.

You don't have to believe this will work for you in order for it to work. You are unlikely to know until you've tried it. Be willing to not know what will happen, and see what unfolds.

NOTES

1   The study was conducted by research analysts Datamonitor and reported in the *Daily Mail*, 19 February 2003.

2   The term 'simple sugars' refers to those carbohydrates with a high 'glycaemic load' (see Chapter 7), and are most commonly overeaten. A substantial amount of research has now accumulated on the addictive nature of food. One science magazine feature provides a summary:

   'A meal loaded up with fat and sugar, it seems, can unhinge the normal hormonal controls that tell people when they are full. Even more intriguing are preliminary findings suggesting that fats and simple sugars can act on the brain in the same way as nicotine and heroin.' From *New Scientist*, February 2003.

   And neuroscientists have discovered that 'the same neural circuitry is involved in the highs and lows of winning money, abusing drugs or anticipating a gastronomical treat'. Reprinted from *Neuron*, 30 (2) Beiter et al, 'Functional Imaging of Neural Responses' 619-39, 2001 with permission from Elsevier.

3   'New knowledge about the brain's reward system, much gained by superrefined brain scanning technology, suggests that as far as the brain is concerned, a reward's a reward, regardless of whether it comes from a chemical or an experience. And where there's a reward, there's the risk of the vulnerable brain getting trapped in a compulsion.' *Science*, 2001; 294: 980-982.

4   From *The Mind and the Brain* by Jeffrey M. Schwartz MD and Sharon Begley (HarperCollins, 2002). Dr Schwartz is Research Professor of Psychiatry at the UCLA School of Medicine.

5   'Association between preference for sweets and excessive alcohol intake.' *Alcohol* 1999; 34: 386-95. However, some preference for sweet and fatty food can be found in almost all animals. In lab tests, when rats are given bread, chocolate, cheese and breakfast cereals instead of their usual plain grains, they overeat and become obese. (Peter J. Rogers,

Institute of Food Research, 'Eating habits and appetite control' *Proceedings of the Nutrition Society* (1999) 58, 59-67.)

6   A major study of the eating habits of 11,000 people over a period of 17 years revealed a significant link between a longer, healthier life and the consumption of fruit. No other food was found to have such a significant effect. Regular fruit eaters had a 24 per cent reduction in death from heart disease, a 32 per cent reduction in deaths from strokes and a 21 per cent reduction in deaths from other causes. Reported in the *British Medical Journal* (1996; 313: 755-779), amended and reproduced with permission from the BMJ Publishing Group. (As for the crisps, see Chapter 7.)

7   Kelly Brownell PhD, Director of the Yale Center for Eating and Weight Disorders, has often been quoted on the subject of the 'toxic environment' we live in today: 'It's like trying to treat an alcoholic in a town where there's a bar every ten feet. Bad food is cheap, heavily promoted, and engineered to taste good.' This is from an article in *National Geographic,* August 2004; Brownell is also interviewed in the documentary *Super Size Me*.

8   A report by the Royal College of Physicians ('Nutrition and Patients', July 2002) found that an alarming 40 per cent of NHS hospital patients were malnourished. As a result, recovery from surgery would be impaired, with a greater risk of infection and more gradual return to normal levels of energy.

CHAPTER 2

Control Your Eating, Not Your Weight

The epidemic of obesity is due to large portions of food eaten by inactive people.
GEORGE BRAY MD, PROFESSOR OF OBESITY, LOUISIANA STATE UNIVERSITY

People *can* change. *Everybody* can. In fact, all of us do change, simply because things happen to us as we go through life that inevitably make an impact and leave us different in some way. The question is not whether we change, but how much we direct change, actively choosing to create the person we really want to be.

There are two crucial things to know about directing this kind of change: it never happens overnight, and it never gets done for you. Change takes time and it takes effort on your part.

However, when it comes to your weight – your body size and shape – it may well be that you've already spent considerable time and effort making changes, but you've found the changes either didn't work or didn't last. This, of course, can leave you doubting your ability to make the changes you want.

If what you tried before was some form of diet, then at

least know you're not alone: the vast majority of people who diet regain all the weight they lose. Maybe that's why you're reading this book. You are looking for something else.

Welcome to a completely different solution. This is not a diet book. This book is about making real, lasting change. The ideas I'll be introducing may not be easy to take on board and use immediately. This doesn't mean they aren't sound or that you are incapable of using them. It just means this will take time.

After all, it took you this long in your life to get to where you are now, so isn't it reasonable to spend some time and effort to make real changes? You may want an easy, instant cure, but is that really possible? What I will show you in these pages is that quick-fix solutions – diets, pills, magic slimming techniques – at best avoid the real problem, and can actually make it worse.

Your Problem isn't Weight

In fact, you may not even be seeing what the real problem is. The chances are you think your problem – what you want to *change* – is your weight. After all, if your body was how you wanted it and stayed that way, would you be reading this book? If you answer 'Of course not!' then here's something for you to consider.

Imagine a smoker who says 'I'm fed up with coughing so much. What can I do to stop my coughing?' Someone points out that it's the smoking that's doing it, but the smoker says 'Yes, I know, but what I really want is some good cough medicine.'

Imagine a problem drinker who says 'My driving is

terrible. I keep having accidents. Where can I get some good driving lessons?' Someone suggests it's because he's driving drunk, so he keeps drinking and takes the bus.

Now, you may know that smokers and drinkers go through periods when they do think like this. It's a kind of denial because they are denying what their problem really is. The difference, though, is that when they finally admit they do have a problem, they tend to see it for what it is. Smokers set out to take control of their smoking, not their coughing. And problem drinkers set out to take control of their drinking, not their driving.

When it comes to eating, though, this step is often not taken, or not taken fully. People who have an addiction to food set out to change a *symptom*: their weight. They keep their sights set on the effect, not the cause, which is eating too much.

The typical overeater says 'I'm two stone overweight, none of my clothes fit properly and I hate how I look. How can I lose weight?' So if someone says 'What you need to do is eat less food' they reply 'I know. I'll join a slimming club.'

You see, your weight is not your problem. It's one of the effects of your problem. Your problem is you eat more food than your body needs. Not more than somebody else's body needs. More than your body needs. Not more than your body used to need when you were younger or more active. More than your body needs now. Not more than your body would need if you had different genes and metabolism. More than your body needs with the genes and metabolism you have. That's why there's extra weight on it.

Saying the problem is 'eating' and not 'weight' might sound at first like I'm just playing with words, but let's think about it because it's very important. *The reason it's important is because the more attached you are to losing weight, the more difficult it will be for you to deal with addictive overeating.* (1)

Let's start to look at why.

The Problems with Weight Loss as Your Goal

Yo-yo Dieting

When weight loss is all you care about, it makes sense to follow a weight-loss diet. But whenever you go on a diet, it's inevitable you'll go off it sooner or later. A diet may help you lose weight, but it's only a temporary solution to a permanent problem: your potential for overeating.

When weight is all you care about, your motivation to eat less disappears along with the weight. When you've lost the weight (or even just some of it) you no longer have any reasons not to overeat. It's only when weight goes back on that you start to think there's a problem. So then you are in that familiar – and unhealthy – cycle of weight loss and gain and loss and gain, known as yo-yo dieting. (2)

Poor Nutrition

When weight loss is all you care about, it's easier to ignore the nutritional value of the food you eat. You may not be giving your body the nutrition it needs, you may even be eating things which do more harm than good, but when weight loss is your priority that's what influences your decisions. You could end up doing things like passing on the beans and rice at dinner because they're 'fattening' but snacking on biscuits later that evening because you fancy them – and after all, you've been so good all day and you're going to work off the extra calories at the gym tomorrow.

This kind of trade-off is typical of those who think entirely in terms of weight. They count calories and drink diet sodas. But watching your weight isn't necessarily the same as watching your health.

An Unhappy Relationship with Food

When weight loss is all you care about, you can end up feeling guilty about eating anything because all food contains calories. Especially after years of calorie-counting, your choices about what to eat can become harder to make because any choice feels like a bad one.

> *A diet may help you lose weight, but it's only a temporary solution to a permanent problem: your potential for overeating.*

An Unhealthy Effect on Your Body

When weight loss is all you care about, your results can be misleading. Weight loss is all too often *lean tissue* loss, which not only ages you prematurely and damages your health, but also makes it even easier to gain excess fat later. On the other hand, if you eat wisely and do even moderate exercise, the lean mass (mostly muscle) you gain can outweigh much of the fat you've lost. This means your *weight* doesn't change as much as your health and appearance does. (3)

Avoiding the Real Problem

When weight loss is all you care about, you avoid facing the reality of your addiction to food. After all, you're not addicted to weight: you don't get cravings late at night for 2lb of fat to add to your thighs.

When weight loss is all you care about, it makes sense to avoid your addictive desire to overeat. If you tend to overeat late at night, for example, you keep yourself busy in the evenings and avoid being alone at home. This has to be a temporary measure, and when the food-addict in you resurfaces, the weight goes right back on because dealing with your addictive eating was never your goal. Weight loss was.

Poor Motivation

When weight loss is all you care about, it's more difficult to stay motivated. There will always be the days when, for various reasons, you just feel 'fat' no matter what you've been eating. Whether this is real or imagined, any sense of success can be short-lived.

When weight loss is your goal and you have a great deal of weight to lose it can feel overwhelming. Having lost 2lb can seem pointless when there's 198 more to go.

When weight loss is your goal you never really achieve it, partly because it's never enough (remember the saying, 'you can never be too rich or too thin') and partly because you fear you won't stay that way. It's such a fragile achievement.

Most important of all, weight loss as a goal makes it easy to disregard the damage overeating does to your health, vitality and to your self-esteem – in ways that have little or nothing to do with how you look. We'll look at this in more detail later.

Why the Problem Can Be So Hard to See

Have you heard the story about someone asking a fish what water is like, and the fish answers 'What's water?' In much the same way, we are swimming around in a culture obsessed with appearances, and it's easy to be so used to it that we simply don't see how much it surrounds us. Just like the fish that takes water for granted, we accept the wrong message – that appearance is all that matters – without question.

This attitude is so common, it's everywhere. When I first started writing this book I would tell friends I was writing a book about *addictive eating*. Everybody who mentioned it again referred to it as a book about *losing weigh*t. I even have a friend who calls it 'your fat book'! And yet people would never call my book on stopping smoking a book about improving lung capacity.

Be careful, because this is very tricky. It might seem simple, but there can be a huge gulf between understanding what I'm saying here and embracing it fully. For example, at this point you might well be thinking that you really do want to deal with your addictive eating. But ask yourself if it's still only a means to one very specific end – to lose weight. Ask yourself how much your priority has to do with your appearance, if you *only* want to control your overeating in order to be a certain size and shape. That's what I'm talking about.

Here's an example. A woman phoned me up to inquire about coming to see me for help. Her eating was out of control and she sounded very distressed about her weight. She wasn't sure whether to see me or join a slimming club much nearer to her home. 'I have a friend who has just lost

28lb with WeightWatchers!' she cried down the phone.
'She's a very old friend!' She was extremely agitated about it
and it was obvious that what had upset her so much was her
friend's weight loss. You know as well as I do that she would
never say, with that same tone of fury in her voice, 'My
friend has been eating a lot less food!' And yet this must be
what the friend had done. My irate caller, like so many
others, was obsessed with the effect instead of the cause.

Take Control of Overeating

Some people do give up their goal of losing weight but they
don't replace it with any other goals with regard to healthy
eating. They just give up doing anything about any of it! You
may identify with this, or it may be you fear this is what will
happen if you let go of your attachment to weight loss as
your goal.

The solution is to understand – *and keep in mind* – how
else you will benefit from taking control of overeating. One
benefit will be weight loss, and, provided you are in fact
overweight, that is an excellent result. However, in order to
do this, you need to make your body size less important to
you and make dealing with your addictive eating your main
goal. This requires a change in your thinking, a shifting of
priorities.

As we will see later on, many different things act together
to create an addictive relationship with food. *One of the most
significant is making your appearance more important to
you than your health.* (4)

Our culture promotes the idea of looking good at all
costs. What matters is having the 'perfect' figure. What

matters less – if at all! – is becoming malnourished through our efforts to achieve it. Anorexia and bulimia are extreme results of this, but it's relevant to all of us to varying degrees. Extra weight is judged, scorned and ridiculed almost everywhere, and encourages us to attach ourselves so strongly and exclusively to the goal of weight loss.

Losing weight is a good consequence of eating less. But when we are preoccupied with our appearance, which is a material concern, we pay less attention to the effects of addictive eating, and what it costs us emotionally and spiritually to be out of control in such a significant area of our lives. And in many insidious ways we take less notice of the cost to our physical health as well.

The point is that while you are overeating, you are holding yourself back from becoming all you could be – in ways that have nothing to do with the size and shape of your body.

If you are like most addicts, you reason that when you have sorted yourself out and become all you can be (whatever that means to you) then you will be able to control your addictive eating. This is putting the cart before the horse. The process of dealing with addictive eating is the path – quite possibly the only path – towards a more confident, peaceful, happier and more fulfilled you. Making positive eating choices for the right reasons can lead you directly towards becoming the person you want to be and living your life the way you really want to live it.

I'm suggesting you pursue a new goal: taking control of your addictive eating because that's your main source of physical and psychological wellbeing. Then losing weight becomes a bonus. It's a very good bonus – assuming you were overweight to begin with – but it's not the focus of everything.

Why it's Vital to Change Priorities

Perhaps by now you are beginning to think 'Yes, but what does it mean to be in control of my eating and how do I do it?' Great! This is a good question to be asking, and you are in the right place to get the answers. Just understand that this is a very different question from 'How do I lose weight?' *The first step in learning to control your addictive eating is to stop asking how you lose weight.*

> **Weight loss as a principal goal is fundamentally flawed.**

This might look like too big a change for you to make. If you are completely preoccupied with wanting to change the shape and size of your body, it may seem impossible to start to care more about your eating. But look at it this way: if you are going on a hundred mile journey due south, and you turn a fraction to the left and take your journey slightly south-east, after a hundred miles you will end up in a very different place. Begin this hundred mile journey by acknowledging that your best goal is to be in control of your overeating. It's actually a journey that will take you the rest of your life, as you are going to be eating – and living in a body of some size and shape – for the rest of your life.

Weight loss as a principal goal is fundamentally flawed. It addresses the effect, not the cause, of your problem, and only one effect at that. It's the one we can all see, but I want to suggest to you it's not even the most important one.

Being in control of your eating has far more significant implications. And wanting to lose weight could be the one thing that keeps you from appreciating what these implications are, because when weight loss is all you care about, you invalidate these other, truly life-enhancing rewards. This is what we will look at further in our next two chapters.

IN OTHER WORDS: TULLIA

I started to have eating problems roughly 15 years ago. I sought help, but because I was not overweight, anorexic or bulimic, nobody would give me help.

I kept on eating junk food even though I had signs of poor health: unpleasant mood swings, PMS, fluid retention, fatigue, frequent nausea and abdominal bloating. I wanted to change but I thought there was no way out. Besides, most of the time I was denying the problem to myself, very much helped by the fact that it was never a weight problem, so I could conceal it.

Once I came to terms with the reality that I was addicted to food, a whole process of change began. I became engaged in a process of self-discovery that has gone far beyond the tangible consequences of overeating.

At first I had a huge resistance to change, yet the more I practise, the more I feel at ease with it and as a consequence with myself.

Taking Control

- Make a list of things you want to change in terms of what and how much you eat. Here are a few examples I've heard from clients: to eat smaller meals; not to snack between meals in the afternoons; not to eat anything after 8pm; to snack on fruit instead of chocolate. Aim to be as specific as possible, so that instead of writing down 'to eat less' you identify what you intend to eat less of and at what time of day or in what circumstances you'll be. You might get some ideas from the list at the beginning of Chapter 1 and from Chapter 7.

- It takes deliberate effort to change your goal from wanting to lose weight to wanting to control your addictive eating, so whenever you think about your weight, think 'Weight is not my problem. Eating is.' This is true whether you are underweight, overweight – or even if you are the weight you want to be.

  If you tend to be very concerned about your weight, it may not at first seem true to think of your problem as 'eating'. This requires a significant change in your thinking. Stay with this, though, because you will find a breakthrough for yourself. Whenever you get caught up in how you look and what you weigh, just remind yourself of any other downside to addictive eating that you regularly experience. Keep reviewing this book and take note of the ways in which changing this emphasis benefits you. There's more about this in the next two chapters.

- If you normally weigh yourself, consider putting your bathroom scales away. I wish you knew how many times I've heard clients say, 'I was doing fine until I got on the scales!!' Unless you have a particular reason for knowing your weight, such as filling in an insurance form or for medical reasons, there's no need to weigh yourself more than once or twice a year, if that.

When you weigh yourself over and over again you are using your weight to see whether you are succeeding or failing. In this book I will show you how to create a different way to gauge success, one which relates to how much you are in control of your eating. In order to take on this new standard, you will need to let go of your old standard.

- You may react to some things in later chapters by thinking: 'But how will that help me to lose weight?' Change your question to: 'How will that help me to take control of my overeating?' and you will see the answer.

- Take special care if you tend to talk a lot with friends or family about weight and dieting. If you regularly discuss these issues, this may be another aspect to your problem because it keeps you focused on the shape and size of your body. Start to think of ways to remove yourself from these conversations. Or, deliberately change the conversation to one about health and nutrition.

NOTES

1   To mention just a couple of studies on this, research conducted at Stanford University School of Medicine (September 1998) found that those women who were the most dissatisfied with their appearance – *whether or not they were overweight* – were the most likely to drop out of diet programmes. And a study at the University of British Columbia (October 2004) showed a strong link between a greater degree of 'body image dissatisfaction' and chronic (yo-yo) dieting.

2   A number of studies have linked yo-yo dieting – where 10 or more pounds are lost three or more times – to poor immune system (University of Washington Medical Center, 2004), lower levels of good, HDL cholesterol (Cedars-Sinai Medical Center, 2001), reduced blood flow to the heart after menopause (University of Michigan, 2003) and increased body weight later in life (University of California at Berkeley, 2004).

3   'Your problem is not excess *weight* so much as it is excess *body fat* coupled with too little muscle . . . it's imperative that you look beyond the simplistic notion of losing weight and concentrate on building muscle at the expense of fat.' From *Biomarkers: The 10 Keys to Prolonging Vitality* by Drs William Evans and Irwin Rosenberg of Tufts University Department of Nutrition and Medicine (Simon & Schuster, 1992). Also see Chapter 7.

4   Eating disorders such as anorexia, bulimia and 'binge eating disorder' are strongly associated with an 'overconcern with appearance'; it's even considered by many to be part of the definition of an eating disorder. It might be useful to look at all difficulties with eating as a matter of degree, and that this could have some relevance to you even though you may not have an 'eating disorder' as such.

CHAPTER 3

All that Glitters...

The stage was my only friend, the only place where I could feel comfortable. It was the one place I felt equal and safe.
JUDY GARLAND

Every day you make choices about food. You may be in a restaurant choosing from a menu, or in a supermarket choosing what to have for dinner that evening. Or you may be standing in your kitchen, trying to decide on a late-night snack before bed. Every day you choose when to eat, what to eat and how much to eat.

In some way, these choices are a problem for you. You eat something and later regret it. You promise yourself not to eat certain kinds of foods but you don't stick to it. You follow a diet for a while but sooner or later find yourself overeating again.

We will look at how to decide when, what and how much to eat in later chapters. First, let's look at another basic factor involved in making these choices: the question of why you might choose either to eat or not to eat something.

Motivation (why am I choosing this?) is crucial as it can make the difference between success and failure in anything you attempt. For example, if I asked you to give me £100, you would most likely want to know why. If I said that in return I'd give you a big smile, you probably wouldn't give me the money. But if I said that in return I'd give you a brand new television, that's more likely to provide you with the motivation, isn't it? In both cases, the action you are taking – giving me £100 – is the same. Without good motivation though, you may not choose to take the action.

When it comes to making changes in your choices about food, there are two fundamentally different ways to motivate yourself:

1 **To improve your appearance** – this includes looking better in your clothes, feeling more confident about how you look, being able to buy a greater range of clothes in the high street, feeling confident enough to go swimming, looking more attractive.
2 **To improve your health and wellbeing** – this includes having more energy, fewer headaches, not feeling so bloated, feeling more relaxed around food, enjoying food more, feeling less guilty or regretful about eating, improved sleep, improved immune system, slowing down the aging process.

Just about everyone will be motivated by a mixture of these two, but what's very common is to have far more interest in the first. For most people, if anything gets them interested in the idea of eating less, it's the image of how much better they're going to look when they've lost some weight. If they end up healthier as well, that's usually thought of as a bonus. (1)

The problem is that there is a world of difference in the

effectiveness of these two kinds of motivation, especially in the longer term.

Most of the books on the market, and of course the slimming clubs, encourage you to concentrate on looking good. But a growing body of evidence is showing that what works best is to prioritise the best possible health.

Award-winning health journalist Susan Clark writes:

> *It may be depressing but it is true that most people who lose weight by restricting their calorie intake put their lost weight – and more – back on. Those who stay trim by eating a healthier diet and adopting a modest exercise programme fare better at keeping the weight off in the long term.* (2)

And top nutritionist Dr Marilyn Glenville writes:

> '*The best kept secret of weight loss and good health is to eat as naturally as possible. Natural foods are the ones your body can digest easily and use to maximum benefit . . . It won't give you the very quick, early weight loss that accompanies so many diets but you will see a gradual reduction in weight which will be far easier to maintain.*' (3)

So, in order to lose weight and keep it off, you make exercise and healthy eating your goal. Simple? Well, not so simple if you are one of those people who are *very* preoccupied with how they look. Whether you are overweight or not, the shape of your body – what you look like – can be your overriding concern, as it is for a great many people, and it's not so easy to let that go in order to make this a *genuine* shift in motivation. The obstacle to making this shift has a great deal to do with self-esteem.

Make Self-esteem Your Goal

Quite simply put, self-esteem is the opinion you have of yourself. It's impossible to have no opinion at all, and even though you may not spend much time thinking about what it is, this opinion has a profound effect on every aspect of your life. Just as the opinion you have of someone else affects every moment you spend with that person, so the opinion you have of yourself affects you.

A poor opinion means you experience low self-esteem, which can lead to persistent feelings of anxiety, insecurity and guilt, even when there's no good reason for these feelings. Positive opinions mean high self-esteem: confidence and ease with oneself, and an ability to accept mistakes and shortcomings as well as compliments and success.

As a general principle, the lower self-esteem a person has, the more they will be attached to how they look, and the less interested they will be in healthy eating for its own sake. On the other hand, people who tend to have higher self-esteem will find it easier to maintain those healthy eating habits that work long term.

It's natural to prefer higher self-esteem, to feel more worthy and capable rather than inadequate and inferior. So when we try to make changes in our lives – going on a diet, for example – one of the main reasons we do it is to feel better, to respect and honour ourselves a bit more. But in trying to feel better, many people make a fundamental mistake. They try to raise their self-esteem by getting approval from other people. All too often we try to prove our worth to others so that we'll feel more worthy inside. And this is not just something we try every now and then; it can become a significant part of our life, our main motivation for doing almost anything at all.

We may try to impress others by owning more things or bigger and better things. Or we may seek approval by working harder, achieving more or by being more caring and helpful. And a great many of us try to impress by looking better – which, of course, means thinner. *Wanting to own a better body can be just as much an attempt to gain self-esteem as is wanting any other possession or achievement that's designed to impress others.*

A great many people want to lose weight primarily to get other people to approve of them more – or at least to avoid their judgement and rejection. It's very common and understandable, but it's got nothing at all to do with building self-esteem. Other people's approval of you is not a bad thing – it's just the wrong place to look for self-esteem. Not only is it the wrong place, it actually contributes to keeping your real self-esteem low.

This is especially true of women because a slim body is what our culture promotes and rewards, but this is relevant to many men, too. The problem is that when improving your appearance is your main – perhaps *only* – motivation behind your eating choices, you will tend to attach less significance to the private sources of genuine self-esteem: your own opinion of you, regardless of what others may think. *And it's the private sources of genuine self-esteem that provide you with much more effective motivation when it comes to taking control of overeating.*

The truth is we are all likely to enjoy looking good. I do too – but I also know a danger lurks in this way of thinking. I call

> **Other people's approval of you is not a bad thing – it's just the wrong place to look for self-esteem.**

it dangerous because it takes me away from my genuine self-esteem and impairs my relationship with food, so it's a kind of motivation I don't deliberately encourage, either in myself or others. It's fairly common for people to do well with their eating for a period of time, lose weight, and then start overeating again because they have become pre-occupied with how they look.

Whether we consider ourselves to be overweight or not, our outward appearance often becomes *all that really matters*. Ask yourself these questions:

- Do you habitually compare your body size to others'?
- Do you feel good about yourself if you turn out to be the slimmest in a group?
- Do you feel bad about yourself if you turn out to be the heaviest in a group?
- Do you form opinions about people based on how fat or slim they are?
- Are you more aware of the calorie content of food than the nutritional content?
- Have you ever thought that if only you were slim you'd be confident and happy – *you would like yourself more?*

It's an illusion a great many of us have bought, *even those who have given up trying to make any changes at all.* And we've bought it quite literally in terms of the products sold to us which promote thinness as a commodity. This is why people literally stake their lives on slimming pills and fad diets, or risk anorexia and bulimia in their struggle for a better sense of self-worth.

Keep in mind, though, that there's no shortage of examples of people who achieved their desired weight loss only to feel, often to their surprise, that this didn't deliver the expected rise in self-esteem. They looked good but inside they knew they still didn't feel so good. We all know the examples of celebrities such as Judy Garland (who was as slim, talented and successful as anyone could ever hope to be) but I bet you know people like this in your own life as well.

Understanding what does and what doesn't build genuine self-esteem is crucial because this affects your daily life. Now. Every time you eat.

When you make choices to eat or not to eat something motivated *primarily* by what you look like, you are thinking in terms of a false sense of self-esteem. If you are considering eating a slice of chocolate cake, for example, and you think 'I won't eat it because it's fattening and I want to fit into my clothes' you are motivating yourself to look good. And when people say 'I will eat it, even though I know it's fattening, because I don't care how I look' *they are still thinking in terms of what other people think of them!* The alternative, of course, is to think in terms of genuine self-esteem – your own opinion of you – and we will get to that later.

Even if you want to lose weight because of poor health, there could still be a strong emotional attachment to your appearance which dominates your motivation. Maybe your doctor *said* 'Lose weight', but what you *heard* was 'You don't look so good in that suit.' And maybe what your doctor really *meant* was 'Get your blood pressure down.'

It could be that now you are thinking 'But *I* like being slim, *I* enjoy it, it pleases *me*.' Yes, I know, I do too, but wanting to be slim may be more about what other people think of you than you realise:

- When you put on weight, isn't it when you think it's going to be noticed by others that your heart sinks?
- When you lose weight, don't you want people to notice, even pointing it out to them if they don't make a comment?
- If you magically became your ideal weight right now, wouldn't you feel thrilled to look at yourself in a mirror? Doesn't a mirror show you what other people see?
- If you magically became your ideal weight right now, would you go to your next social event in the shapeless clothes you keep for when you're fat?

Weight and appearance have been so overemphasised in our culture, it's almost impossible not to be affected by it – especially for women. Think of every film you ever saw, where the skinniest, tiniest women are the central, most interesting characters. Look at any mannequin in any shop window. Look at all our fashion models who live dangerously close to starvation. Does this make any sense? It makes sense if you are in the business of selling false self-esteem. Then it makes very good sense, because there is no shortage of buyers.

Losing weight can create a temporary 'high' in the same way as buying a flashy car or wearing the latest fashion does. That high can be powerful and *very* seductive, but inside nothing's changed, and you know it. Nothing can fool the truth inside your own heart, and in your own heart you know that having a more impressive body does nothing to improve your genuine self-esteem. As the old saying goes, all that glitters isn't gold.

It may be you have already figured this out and stopped trying to lose weight. You may be well aware that the image you present to the world does little to improve the image you have of yourself. And you may genuinely esteem yourself in ways that have nothing to do with what you eat.

But still, you may have missed a very exciting opportunity. This is the opportunity to make changes in your eating, not to impress others, but in order to live your life to the full. Not so much because you *look* your best, but because you *feel* your best – because you have higher *genuine* self-esteem. *You could regard your choices about eating as the way to raise your genuine self-esteem. If you do that, you may benefit in more ways than you can imagine.*

Shifting the Balance

Your appearance will no doubt always be significant to you, as mine is to me. I'm not suggesting for one minute that you should no longer care about what you weigh and have no thoughts at all about what your body looks like. What I'm talking about is putting all that into a different perspective, shifting the balance so you give more attention to private sources of health and genuine self-esteem. The more you concern yourself with improving your own opinion of you – regardless of your weight – the more you will be able to stay in touch with motivation *that really works.* (4)

Here's a way to think about it. Imagine that a wicked fairy has put a magic curse on you so that you are never going to lose any weight, and your body is always going to look exactly as it does now. The big question is, *would you have any other reasons to change your eating?*

I'm not suggesting that you won't lose weight or that you shouldn't want to lose weight. What I'm suggesting is *how* to lose the weight – and how to maintain it. It's simply that making this switch in the emphasis of your motivation *works*. The reason it works is because your self-esteem is enhanced when you place the emphasis of your motivation on supporting your health and wellbeing. Psychologically, this is worlds apart from being primarily concerned with your appearance.

Here's a common example. Some people struggle with their weight for years, and then one day they have a health crisis, such as a heart attack. It's a big wake-up call and all of a sudden they switch their motivation from looking good to *staying alive*. They make major changes in their eating, lose the weight and keep it off. This is because they start to prioritise their health. They are also prioritising their self-esteem because they realise how much they don't want to be the sort of person who destroys their own health like that. The point is that you can do this in a preventative way – so you don't have to wait until you have a heart attack!

If you tend to have low self-esteem, you might be thinking 'If only I felt better about myself, then I would make changes in my eating.' Just understand you've got it the wrong way round. People with low self-esteem can make huge changes – and gain a very exciting and powerful sense of self-esteem as a result. I know this because I have seen so many of my clients go through this process. You may struggle initially because you're convinced you'll fail, but it's exactly in the facing of this fear that strength and confidence in yourself will arise.

Or, you might object to the idea of raising your level of self-esteem at all. Some people make the mistake of thinking that high self-esteem is an arrogant, inflated opinion of oneself, self-obsession and indifference to others. This is *not* self-esteem; in fact it is a lack of genuine self-esteem that leads people to become so self-important. Feeling superior is just another false esteem fix.

Or, you could be someone who tends to have high self-esteem already, who rarely feels any need to prove their worth to others. This is a good place to start from, but don't assume you won't benefit from taking control of overeating. It could be that you maintain strong self-esteem from your relationships and from creative and satisfying work. This can distract you from a degree of self-loathing with regard to your physical self, at least for much of the time. Making a change here, though, can certainly bring an immensely rewarding dimension to your life.

Genuine self-esteem comes from within; it's private.

I find the words 'inner joy' helpful in describing genuine self-esteem. Can you honestly say you wouldn't want more of that? It doesn't mean you will never make mistakes. It means you won't feel quite so crushed when you do. It doesn't mean you'll feel instantly confident in facing new challenges. It means you're more likely to appreciate both the challenge and yourself for facing it. Most of all, it doesn't rely on other people applauding your achievements. That's nice when it happens, but it's not essential.

Genuine self-esteem comes from within; *it's private.* This means you improve it at the same time as you let go of some of the significance of what other people might think of you. Work towards making your self-esteem more important to you and the appearance of your body a bit less important. Then you are shifting the balance of these two kinds of motivation.

This still leaves the question of how to improve your genuine self-esteem, so in the next chapter we'll see what a leading authority on self-esteem has to say. This is just one view of many on this subject. I present you with this approach because I know it works, especially when it comes to taking control of addictive eating. My suggestion is to try it and see if it works for you.

IN OTHER WORDS: VANESSA

I've had a weight problem since my early teens. I've gone to a couple of different slimming clubs many, many times and I've had years of therapy. None of it worked. At best, I lost the weight but immediately put it all on again. I've had quite serious periods of depression, which were in very large part due to my weight.

I used to think to myself over and over again, 'You're fat. You're disgusting. You can't eat.' That's what would go on in my head, all the time. It was so negative, and always I'd be eating and eating. I would have conversations with my mother, especially during my 20s, when she would tell me, basically, 'You're obese and your boyfriend will leave you for a slimmer woman.' I'm not sure I was obese, but I'm sure I thought I was fatter than I really was. If I was asked to point out someone who was the same size as me (and I have done this with my boyfriend) I would point to someone who was three times larger.

My mother (who has always been slim) thought that if only I was slimmer I'd be happier. This was probably true, but the way she talked to me about it made me feel so bad about myself.

I was still very overweight when my boyfriend ➤

proposed to me. You might think that the image of myself as a bride in eight months' time would have given me good motivation to lose weight, but over the next month after getting engaged I ate so much I put on another stone. I didn't stop eating, just because I was so focused on how I was going to look as a fat bride. I felt wound up, panicked and I was eating and eating and eating.

What changed for me after doing the course with Gillian was being able to look at the bigger picture. I realised that nobody was marrying me because I'm slim anyway, and that part of the plan was to have children as soon as possible. So I changed my motivation from 'what will I look like on my wedding day?' to 'how can I get myself as healthy as possible to go through the process of having children in my late 30s?'

I have never looked at it like that before, the difference between what I look like and how healthy I am. So I'm learning about nutrition and trying lots of new recipes. I've got out books I bought years ago and never read, and I'm learning how to cook in different ways, with less salt and less fat. I've been buying a lot less processed food and white bread. I had a couple of pieces of toast a few weeks ago and felt so sleepy afterwards I almost fell asleep on the couch. It was incredible.

I'm eating smaller portions by using the techniques from the course. I'm finding learning about nutrition fascinating and I'm discovering lots of information on the Internet. I'm eating a lot of things I never used to eat before and my diet is much more varied. I used to eat the same things over and over again, whether I was on a diet ➤

or not, and it was quite boring. Now I'm not abstaining from anything in particular, I'm never hungry and I've lost weight, although I'm seeing that as a side-effect. It's not what I'm concentrating on, because if I was I'd be back at square one.

My eyes and hair are shiny, my skin is clear. Someone came up to me recently and told me I looked radiant. I'm less tired and have much more energy. And I'm happier than I've been in a long time. I've calmed down about the whole thing and I feel relaxed.

I always used to tell myself that I was going to have a weight problem all my life. But now I think, no, I'm not always going to have a weight problem. I'm going to be healthy and that's what I really want to do.

Taking Control

- List, with as much detail as you can, how it benefits you to be in control of your addictive eating and what it costs you to be out of control. Put the emphasis on health and wellbeing, rather than appearance. Keep the list somewhere safe, private and easily accessible, like a Filofax, diary or jewellery box. Refer to it often, adding to it as you go along. These are notes to yourself in the future, if you forget.

- If you motivate yourself entirely with the goal of weight loss, when the weight is lost the motivation often gets lost as well. When you are at your target weight, you have arrived and it can seem that there's very little reason not to eat in an addictive way. To counteract this, *start out* by placing value on the more private achievements: any benefit you get from eating less other than losing weight. These benefits will be relevant no matter what you weigh. If you can't think of any, you'll find some ideas in the next chapter and in Chapter 7.

- Whenever you think about your weight (for example, if you see yourself in a photo, anticipate a big social event or try on clothes that do or don't fit) deliberately recall these other benefits.

- When you lose weight, don't mention it to anyone. If anyone makes a comment, just let it go and change the subject if possible. The more you get caught up in your improved appearance, the more you upset the balance of your motivation – and the less likely your weight loss will last!

- If you are getting support with your eating issues from a group or a counsellor, resist mentioning, discussing and especially applauding weight loss.

- If you tend to buy smaller clothes with the intention of slimming into them, you encourage yourself to stay focused on your appearance, and this will get in your way.

- If you are one of those people who compares their body size and shape to others, the next time you notice yourself doing this, remind yourself that your self-esteem has nothing to do with the size of someone else's body.

- Are you really overweight? There's a huge difference between wanting to lose weight because your size indicates that you are at risk of serious illness and wanting to lose weight to become fashionably slim. If you are already within the healthy weight range, if you already eat in a healthy way, and if you are reading this book purely because you want to be even slimmer, then you could be creating a problem for yourself, both in terms of health and your addictive relationship with food.

There is, however, some controversy about what is a healthy weight range. Officially, we are overweight if we have a body mass index (BMI) over 25, but some people say that we can be just as healthy with a BMI of 26 or 27. The reason for this confusion is at least partly because BMI does not take into account the proportion of lean mass to body fat; it's a high percentage of body fat that indicates poor health, not simply *weight*.

NOTES

1   One survey (reported in the *Times*, 14 October 2004) found that a mere 23 per cent of those who wanted to lose weight did so *mainly* for health reasons.

2   From *What Really Works* by Susan Clark (Thorsons, 2000).

3   From *Natural Alternatives to Dieting* by Marilyn Glenville, PhD (Ted Smart, 1999).

4   In *Make The Connection* (Century, 1996) Oprah Winfrey and Bob Greene have written a beautiful passage about this which explains their title. Unfortunately, these few sentences are overshadowed by a preoccupation with appearance for the rest of the book:

   'The connection is a change in perception. It is first realising that losing weight is not what is most important. Instead, the excess weight is merely a symptom of a larger problem and losing weight is a side effect, a nice one certainly, of something much more important. It is really about increasing self-confidence, inner strength, and discipline. It is about feeling better on a daily basis, having control over your life, and caring about yourself. Ultimately it is about self-love.

   '[When you've made the connection] you will want only the best for you, which means exercising and eating right, as well as dealing with your problems in a healthy way. You will know you've made the connection when you care enough about yourself that you don't consider doing anything outside your best interest.'

CHAPTER 4

Motivation that Works

No one can make you feel inferior without your consent.
ELEANOR ROOSEVELT

Dr Nathaniel Branden is a psychologist who has been investigating the significance of self-esteem for about 40 years. He has written about 16 books on the subject, many of which are bestsellers and published in a number of languages. In *The Six Pillars of Self-Esteem* (1) he describes the six principles on which self-esteem depends:

1 living consciously
2 self-acceptance
3 self-responsibility
4 self-assertiveness
5 living purposefully
6 personal integrity

These are not just ideas, they are ways to live. Not as ideal states of perfection – that is unrealistic – but as directions to aim towards. The more you live by these principles, the higher your self-esteem will be. And in our relationship with food, *it is exactly the practice of these six principles that gives us the ability to take control of addictive eating.* In fact, I can't think of one thing we need to do in order to take control of an addiction that isn't on that list. When we apply these principles to our addictive behaviour, we take control and we raise our self-esteem at the same time.

Living Consciously

Setting out to live more consciously means that you are open to learning and discovering. Do you know that the word 'curiosity' comes from the same root as the word 'cure'? Your curiosity leads you to your cure. It's doing it right now! It's not sufficient, however, simply to be curious; *living* consciously implies that what you discover gets put into practice.

Although nobody can be conscious of everything all the time, in general, the more aware you are the greater your ability to change. As a simple example, if you want to cut down on sugar you will do better if you're aware of which foods contain sugar.

Many aspects of addictive behaviour become automatic so that we are simply unaware of what's happening. It may be, at times, that you aren't even aware that you are eating. As you become more conscious, you get more control. Each chapter in this book will help you understand more about addictive eating, and will therefore bring you greater ability to take conscious control – and, as a direct result, raise your self-esteem.

Self-acceptance

Learning to accept yourself *doesn't* mean you think everything's perfect just as it is. What it means is that you become your own friend, not your enemy. Even though you dislike many things about being addicted to food, have some compassion for the human being who is caught up in it. It's recognising your inherent worth as a human being – *regardless of anything you do and regardless of what you look like* – that inspires you to create a way of life that reflects and honours you.

Self-acceptance also means accepting that things are the way they are. Accept that, at least sometimes, you eat in an addictive way. Accept that it's impossible for you to continue to eat that way and maintain the best possible state of health. Accept that these things are true, no matter how much you may dislike them.

Self-responsibility

You practise the principle of self-responsibility when you acknowledge that you're the one who's in charge of you. For example, I am not in charge of what you do, so everything in the book is completely, totally, absolutely up to you to use or not. That might seem obvious, but before you can really take it on board, you need to know that you don't *have to* make any changes at all. Ever.

Taking responsibility gives you an extraordinary degree of control because it brings you the freedom to choose. *Taking responsibility is a step towards freedom, not away from it.* In Chapter 5 we will explore this much further, how to make it real and how to put it into practice.

Whenever you achieved something, it's because you took responsibility for it. Perhaps you can think of things you've accomplished simply because you stopped waiting for something to happen to take care of it for you. You paid off a debt. You finished a household project. You left a bad job.

Perhaps you can remember the empowering effect this had on your self-esteem.

Self-assertiveness

There will be times when you'll want to assert yourself to others about what you are or are not going to eat. It makes a big difference if you can start to make your own choices, at least sometimes, instead of always eating what other people want you to eat, or eating something simply because everyone else is.

You may want to practise asserting yourself when people push you to eat when it's really not right for you to do so. You may need to talk with the person who shops and cooks for you, in order to make clear agreements about what you want.

It can be a very big step to say 'no thanks' when something's offered, or to order a salad while your friends have pizza. There will be times when it might not be appropriate to do so, but when you do assert yourself in this way, notice the effect it has on your private sense of self-esteem.

Living Purposefully

It's important to have some kind of intention to make changes, to choose goals and work towards achieving them. This is living purposefully – although it's not our achievements that enhance self-esteem as much as the process we engage in on our way.

A sense of purpose about food provides us with a direction, and without a direction we are very likely to get lost. We will be too easily led by whims, aimless and even chaotic.

If you've followed the 'Taking Control' section at the end of Chapter 2, you've already started setting some goals of your own. By all means let go of your specific weight-loss goals, but you won't achieve much if you don't replace them with goals about taking control of addictive eating. As you read on you'll find more goals you can aim for in every chapter.

Personal Integrity

Any time your actions don't fit with your principles, your personal integrity will suffer, and so will your self-esteem. After all, if another person lied to you, damaged your health or made you do things you later regretted, you wouldn't hold them in very high esteem, would you? When it comes to food, you may

> *You take control of addictive eating and you raise your self-esteem at the same time.*

have been doing this to yourself in many ways for a long time. To take a common example, many people will buy family-sized packs of snacks 'for the children', only to eat them all themselves. They lie to themselves, and their self-esteem suffers as a result.

Even if you get just a bit more honest with yourself, your sense of personal integrity will soar and so will your self-esteem. It simply means doing what you believe in, doing what you say you will do, and telling the truth to yourself. When it comes to food, do not put up with lies, or even 'white lies' such as 'oh, just this once'. Addictive behaviour is always maintained by deceptions of various kinds. Telling the truth is your way out. You take control of addictive eating and you raise your self-esteem at the same time.

These six principles may well be familiar to you, and not only in connection with eating. And it may well be that you have practised these principles and enjoyed the benefits of healthier self-esteem when you've been in control of your eating in the past. But it may also be that your improved appearance was all that really mattered, so you invalidated and ignored these sources of genuine esteem. The value in declaring your self-esteem as the main motivation behind choices about eating is that the process is more deliberate. It is therefore more powerful and effective.

Whether you recognise it or not, every time you make a choice about eating there is an effect on your self-esteem. With a single choice the effect is likely to be subtle, but the extraordinary thing about food is that you encounter it all the time, so you affect your self-esteem all the time. The effect is constant and cumulative.

Higher self-esteem is something you can achieve, and your relationship with food provides you with a unique opportunity to achieve it. Your self-esteem is affected by all aspects of your life, but food has a very special significance. Not only is food a regular part of your daily life – it's also fundamental and essential. Your food becomes you – so what and how much you eat has a more profound effect on your self-esteem than almost anything else.

Your Rewards

Learning that *you* determine your opinion of yourself and that you have an enormous impact on your self-esteem daily may at first seem both liberating and frightening. Many people believe that self-esteem is an inevitable consequence of childhood; that if they were invalidated by parents and teachers when they were young, they must resign themselves to low self-esteem for life. They are self-critical and believe that whatever they do, it's never enough.

Self-esteem does have its roots in the past, but it *is* possible for you to change. The only thing that could prevent you is your fear of the very changes you want to make. Your fear of change may sound familiar: 'Oh, but this is me – it's just how I am!' Remember to go as slow or as fast as you want; it's not a race. Get support if you want to. You have the rest of your life to work on this, and even small steps can produce exciting results.

Not only does your relationship with food improve, but by applying these principles to eating, you also increase their significance in your life. In taking control of your addictive eating you take more control of your life in general. By becoming more at peace with your eating you become more at peace with yourself. In gaining a healthy relationship with food you improve your relationships with everyone – especially yourself.

And for many people, raising your self-esteem will be the only way you can make 'looking good' lose some of its significance. You may have believed for much of your life that your worth as a person is determined by the size of your body, and you'll find that things really start to change when you give up trying to establish your self-worth in this way. Since it doesn't generate genuine self-esteem anyway, *it's never enough*, even when you do receive some form of approval from others for how you look.

This is an arena that provides you with opportunities like no other. Begin by treating yourself as if you are more worthy, regardless of your size, and before too long you will feel more worthy, regardless of your size. *Simply pay attention to all the ways your life improves when you are in control of your eating:*

Benefits You Gain from Raising Your Level of Self-esteem

▌ inner strength and confidence, rather than feeling like a victim of life

▌ inner joy and peace, which is less dependent on external circumstances

▌ feeling more at ease with yourself, either when you're alone or with others

▌ feeling grounded and centred

▌ productivity and enthusiasm for life

▌ less dependent and therefore more satisfying relationships

▌ greater ability to trust yourself and your own thinking

▌ creativity, because you believe in yourself more

▌ less sensitive to criticism

▌ less self-conscious and anxious

▌ more positive mood, less depressed

▌ decreased need to be defensive, competitive or judgemental

▌ greater ability to recover from other compulsive behaviours such as smoking

▌ greater ability to cope with major life changes, such as the death of a relative, the end of a relationship, redundancy or retirement

Benefits You Gain, Besides Higher Self-esteem and Weight Loss

- you take control of your life instead of being controlled by your addictive appetite
- greater enjoyment of eating, free from guilt, regrets, fear or anxiety
- vitality and sustained energy, feeling more alive
- more emotionally balanced, improved mood
- social life free from preoccupation with food
- freedom from bloated, uncomfortable feelings from eating too much
- freedom from dieting
- freedom to cook anything for others, knowing you don't have to eat it
- ability to think more clearly, better concentration and attention span
- savings in money and time
- more adaptable to temperature changes
- less susceptible to symptoms of stress
- improved sleep
- better health

I could list all the health issues connected with addictive eating, but the truth is there aren't many that are not affected by the food we eat. It's crucial to acknowledge that the ongoing maladies you may suffer from – such as fatigue, infections, headaches, constipation, diarrhoea, haemorrhoids, premenstrual tension, stomach aches, bad complexion and clogged sinuses – are in almost all cases preventable and treatable by the quality and quantity of the food you eat. Even serious conditions such as high blood pressure, late-onset diabetes, heart disease, strokes, osteoporosis, arthritis and cancer are in many cases directly linked with addictive eating. (2)

Many people believe these illnesses are determined by the luck of their genes, and it is true that we do tend to inherit the same genetic 'Achilles' heel' as other members of our family. What this means, though, is that addictive eating in one family usually leads to diabetes, while in another family it usually leads to heart disease or a particular kind of cancer. In another, arthritis, and so on.

By taking control of your addictive eating you will at the very least delay the onset of these conditions, and you could avoid them altogether. Many factors work together to create illness: stress, genes, inactivity, environment, age. Certainly our minds and emotions play no small part. Food is also a very significant factor – and as an addicted eater this may well be the last thing you want to acknowledge.

Have we strayed off the subject of self-esteem here? No. When you value your physical health, your self-esteem is strengthened, just as eating in a way that harms your health undermines it.

How Not to Sabotage Yourself

Even after all this, I suspect I still haven't fully convinced you. I am well aware of the allure of 'looking good'. If you think you could look like a film star, and I'm just offering you self-esteem, what are you most likely to use to motivate yourself? You might just bargain 'Okay, okay, I'll go for the self-esteem if it will help me lose all this dreadful weight'!

The attraction of weight loss as your main goal can be

even stronger if you are very overweight. You may not want to look like a star, just a 'normal' person who doesn't get rude stares everywhere they go. Even so, prioritising weight loss will lead you off track.

You might lose some weight, but chances are you will sabotage yourself in some way if your self-esteem remains low. People who dislike themselves often punish themselves by doing things they know they will regret later on. Then this self-destructive behaviour lowers their self-esteem even more. You may be all too familiar with 'I'm fat, so I'm worthless, so I might as well eat more, so I overeat, then I feel guilty, and I get fatter, which proves I'm worthless, so I might as well eat . . .'

This vicious circle is driven by exaggerated, inappropriate guilt, which is the hallmark of low self-esteem. In the past you may have tried to break this cycle by trying to lose weight. But if you measure your worth by your body size, it may be a long time before you feel any better about yourself, so it's easy to return to overeating. Weight loss is slow, but you can benefit from applying the 'Six Pillars' almost immediately.

You can apply the practice of the 'Six Pillars' – living consciously, self-acceptance, self-responsibility, self-assertiveness, living purposefully and personal integrity – specifically to food, whatever your appearance. You break the cycle by raising your self-esteem. And when you apply these principles to your eating, your self-esteem will improve long before you achieve any significant weight loss.

In order to do this, though, you need to start by stressing motivation that is about anything other than your weight, shape and size. *Look for any reason to make changes in your eating other than your appearance.*

When I keep in mind the impact my eating has on my self-esteem, I don't overeat because I know the rewards are precious. I become significantly happier, regardless of external circumstances in my life. I can't think of anything else that has as much impact on my self-esteem as my eating. Not my weight. My *eating*.

> *To make lasting changes, you'll need to find more pleasure in controlling your eating than in overeating. Otherwise you won't stay with it.*

That's what works for me. Just try it, and see if it works for you. If it doesn't, you can discard it. It doesn't have to be a permanent commitment.

The truth is that you are much more likely to control your addictive overeating if you are going to get something you really want out of it. Whether it's drinking, smoking, overeating or whatever, the most compelling aspect of any addiction is that it brings you pleasure. If you try to limit this pleasure in order to please or impress others, it becomes an act of self-sacrifice, and it's impossible to stay motivated to keep sacrificing yourself. Not only that, but your motivation is dependent on how others are treating you. If they ever let you down, the thing to do for yourself will be to return to addictive eating. To make lasting changes, you'll need to find more pleasure in controlling your eating than in overeating. Otherwise you won't stay with it.

IN OTHER WORDS: JULIET

I have struggled with eating issues for many years, trying to deal with them via various diets and nutritional schemes and also different types of counselling. In the past, these struggles were to do with both the quality of the food I ate, as well as the quantity.

Over the years, I began to eat more organic food. There were still the occasional 'blow-outs', but overall my diet featured lots of fruit and vegetables, wholemeal bread, etc. Anybody looking at me from the outside would have thought that I was eating sensibly and healthily. However, the issue of how much I ate remained problematic. I could never shake off my concern that I needed to tackle portion size and frequency of meals.

When I found Gillian's book, I instantly knew that her message of eating less was what I had been looking for. Having said that, the idea of eating less was scary, all the more so as the diet industry has tried to find diets and foodstuffs which allow people to be slim and healthy while eating as much as they like. This quest is of course embedded in our culture where unchecked consumption, whether in the form of food or consumer goods, has come to be seen as a right. Satiation and 'having (eaten) enough' are virtually impossible to achieve, especially as large amounts of money are invested in product development, marketing and advertising in order to permanently create new desires.

We expect to be able to consume to our heart's content, and when this then manifests itself in, for ➤

example, too much body fat, we want an easy and painless instant fix. Gillian's message is a simple one, yet it is not an easy one! It certainly does get easier, though, and the permanent cycle of dieting and bingeing, with its accompanying cycle of hope and despair, was incredibly difficult and painful to endure. The challenge laid out by Gillian to eat less is a constructive one, whereas the dieting and subsequent over-feeding are purely destructive. The false promise that we can eat all we want and maintain good health is not sustainable for our bodies, and neither is it sustainable for the planet. Deciding to eat less is a very profound and challenging step. This is the only technique I have come across which has worked for me in a way that lasts. Less is more!

Taking Control

- Whenever you eat in an addictive way, be brave enough to do it in front of other people just as much as you do it on your own. This will help you to lessen the significance of other people's opinions of you when it comes to your relationship with food. It's not that other people's opinions aren't important, it's just that it damages your own self-esteem if you make their opinions of you more important than your own.

- Don't tell other people about your achievements in taking control of your addictive eating. By keeping this to yourself you begin to break down some of your dependency on other people's approval. Get used to feeling *your* pride in *your* accomplishments, acknowledging the effect on your own self-esteem – privately.

- Identify and stay in touch with benefits other than weight loss and you have much more powerful and immediate feedback which will keep you motivated. Focusing on weight loss alone can be discouraging if you have a lot of weight to lose because your end result seems such a long way off. Instead, you can say, 'Okay, I still don't look so great, but at least I'm in control and I'm eating in a way that supports my health and self-esteem.' And that's *something*!

- When you do lose some weight, it's inevitable and very understandable that you'll feel delighted. However, this is exactly the time when you need to be extra cautious. Your addictive eating is likely to resurface if you don't keep a good balance of motivation, so remind yourself of the health and self-esteem benefits you are getting. It will help you a great deal to resist wearing clothes that emphasise your new shape and size, at least for a while. I'm not suggesting you should never wear smaller sizes; I'm suggesting you take things very slowly. Changing your body shape is a big thing to do. Ease into it gradually, make it as insignificant as you possibly can, and it's much more likely to last.

- It can be helpful to realise that low self-esteem is often behind the moods you might think of as 'having a bad day', 'feeling negative' or 'hating my life'. At times like this you may tend to think 'if only I was slimmer, all my problems would disappear'. Strengthening your self-esteem may not make all your problems disappear, but it will come a lot closer to it than losing weight will!

NOTES

1   From *The Six Pillars of Self-Esteem* by Nathaniel Branden, PhD (Bantam, 1994).

2   'Possibly the greatest misconception people have about the process of aging is that it's synonymous with illness. There are two principal factors responsible for the onset and severity of most chronic and degenerative conditions – your genetic heritage, which you cannot control; and your lifestyle, which you can and should control.' From a book written by two professors of nutrition and medicine at Tufts University: *Biomarkers: The 10 Keys to Prolonging Vitality* by Drs Evans and Rosenberg (Simon & Schuster, 1992).

   And from *Healing: Without Freud or Prozac* by Dr David Servan-Schreiber of the University of Pittsburgh School of Medicine (Macmillan UK, 2003): '... a revolution that is still in the making: the scientific demonstration that nutrition has a profound impact on practically all the leading causes of disease in Western societies'.

CHAPTER 5

Set Yourself Free

There is no must in art because art is free.
WASSILY KANDINSKY

Over the two decades that I've been teaching this material, I've very rarely met anyone with a really good sense of choice about the changes they wanted to make. Almost everyone starts out by denying choice to some extent – *and this is in very large part why they struggle so much.*

On the other hand, I've seen over and over again that when people start to engage with this notion of choice, things really start to happen. So much falls into place, and it puts everything in a completely new context. In this chapter we'll look at how you can do this.

First, let's look at a situation in which you wouldn't be eating addictively, but where you wouldn't have a choice about it. Imagine for a moment what it would be like if somebody else was in control of your food, deciding when, what and how much you eat. They give you just enough food to stay healthy and no more, and you don't have access to anything else to eat. Of course this could only be done if they had restrained you in some way, if you were locked up in a cell from which there was no escape.

Otherwise you'd be free to run off and eat whatever you fancied.

How do you think you'd react in that situation? My guess is you would have a mixture of two completely different reactions. One would be compliance, and the other would be some kind of rebellion.

Compliance means you go along with the way things are, even feeling grateful for being locked up because finally you are not overeating. You try your best to conform and to 'be good'.

Rebellion could take many different forms. You might be rude and uncooperative towards your gaolers. You might get depressed or irritable. You might spend all your time thinking of a way to get out – by becoming ill, for example. Your rebellion would be fuelled by your anger and resentment over the injustice of not being free to eat whatever you wanted. You might become completely obsessed with all the foods you can't have. And when you were finally let out, you'd most likely devour them by the bucketful. This is what you might call 'being bad'.

Different personalities will identify with one of these reactions more than the other, but the chances are you would experience them both in varying degrees as time went on. On one day in your cell you might feel relieved and secure, thinking: 'this is great, look at all the weight I'm losing'. But on another day all you would think about is your favourite 'comfort foods' and how much you wanted them and missed them – especially if you could smell them and see other people eating them!

This scenario illustrates how you are affected by how much you own your choices about what you eat. If you are locked up in the cell as I just described, you aren't making any choices about the quantity or quality of the food you eat. Your jailer is. The point is that whenever people try to eat less, they invariably mimic this situation in their minds. They create a mental attitude that imitates being locked up in a cell with only enough food to survive. This is because they deny choice.

Most people fear that if they have the freedom to overeat, they will.

In large part, this creates the cycle of alternately dieting and bingeing that so many people find themselves caught up in. They lock themselves into a diet, comply with its restrictions for as long as they can, then make up for lost time as soon as they've been 'released'. They might decide they've been released when they've reached their target weight. Or they might decide it's when they've broken the diet, at a party perhaps. Once they are out of that cell, they feel compelled to overeat and hardly stop. And it's – very understandably – a long, long time before they are going to get themselves back into that cell again.

Whether you've ever followed diets or not, the chances are you can identify with this to some degree. Maybe you say to yourself 'I *can't* have any more' or 'that's *forbidden*'. Or 'I'm *not allowed* to eat anything with sugar in' or 'I *mustn't* eat between meals' or 'I've *got to* stop eating so much'. Most people fear that if they have the freedom to overeat, they will. *So in order to take control they must deny themselves that freedom.*

With thoughts like these, there's only one way to go: comply for as long as you can, and then rebel. Compliance will look like control, but the prohibitive thinking means that it will often feel like deprivation. Eventually, even the thought of compliance feels like deprivation, which is why many people overeat just before starting a diet. *This is a very big part of addictive eating. It's eating more food than you need so that you don't feel deprived.*

But how much you feel deprived has very little to do with how much you are or are not eating. I'm not talking about physical deprivation in the sense of famine, malnutrition or starvation. The feelings of deprivation we're looking at here come from your attitude, the way you are thinking. That state of mind is one of resentment created by believing you are prohibited – or prohibiting yourself – from eating something, that you are restricted or bound by certain rules. It's created from thinking things like 'I have to', 'I must', 'I'm not allowed', 'I can't' and 'I never will again'.

Bad choices are still choices, and that's the crucial point.

Here's one example of how this works that happened to me recently. I was looking at some leaflets – the kind available at the doctors' – to see what was the official advice on nutrition these days. One of these leaflets was about keeping your heart in good shape, and it listed foods that contribute to heart disease. On this list was 'pork pies'. I read it and then forgot all about it. I'm not a big pork pie eater; I probably have something like one or two a year. But a few days later in the supermarket I found myself drawn to a shelf full of – you guessed it – pork pies! I really wanted one, but I was also curious about this sudden interest in something I don't usually buy. Then I remembered the leaflet. Without realising, I had mentally recorded pork pies as 'forbidden' and the rebel in me showed up as predictably as day follows night.

If I had then reacted by telling myself 'don't you dare eat

one of those!' I would have made things worse, because then I would have wanted one even more. Instead, I gave myself permission to eat all the pork pies I wanted – remembering what the consequences of doing so would be. I gave myself a choice. I do believe that eating pork pies every day would be a series of bad choices. But bad choices are still choices, and that's the crucial point.

The position I take is 'This is my body and it's up to me what goes in it. I'm in charge here. Health experts give me helpful information, but I choose whether or not I follow their advice.'

If I don't take that step, all I can do is rebel – or comply for a while and then rebel all the more! *The more I recognise my freedom to choose, the less I feel deprived and the less I need to rebel.* When it comes to taking control of addiction, it makes all the difference when people genuinely acknowledge the free choices available to them. *This is the key: own your choices and, as a result, you take control.*

Signs of Denial of Choice

Language – 'I mustn't eat any more cake.'

In order to use this information, you'll need to become aware of the language you use, both in your private thoughts and when you speak to others. What sort of things do you say to yourself? Do you use prohibitive language? Diets inevitably include a list of 'forbidden' or 'banned' foods, and diet books tell you what you are 'allowed' to eat, what you 'can't' eat and what you 'must not' or 'have to' do. If you aren't aware of this language and the powerful effect it has,

DEPRIVATION OR CHOICE

If you try to eat less by telling yourself:

I can't . . . I mustn't . . . I shouldn't . . . I won't . . .
I have to stop . . . I've got to stop . . . I'm not allowed . . .
I'm not able to . . . it's forbidden . . . I never will again . . .

*You'll react as if
you were locked up
and forced to eat less:*

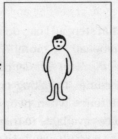

Either you comply:
Be good and follow the rules
Eat less food
Feel happy and grateful
Don't eat junk food
Lose weight
Feel relieved and successful
Feel less hungry

Or you rebel:
Feel deprived, angry, resentful
Feel miserable, depressed,
   martyred
Can't stop thinking about food
Feel guilty about eating
Eat compulsively whenever
   a good excuse comes along
Feel more hungry

*Compliance looks good – but it leads to rebellion
sooner or later!*

The solution is to tell yourself:

THIS IS MY CHOICE
I CAN EAT ANYTHING I WANT
I CAN EAT AS MUCH AS I WANT

- Say these things to yourself whenever you think about eating something, while you are eating and when you've finished – *especially* if it's addictive eating.
- Fear of failure makes free choice difficult to grasp. The fear is: 'If I really can eat anything I want, I know I will.' Then, what follows is denial of free choice in an attempt to eat less.
- You've always got free choices, no matter what the consequences of those choices may be. A bad choice is still a choice. With each choice, either to eat or not to eat something, you choose: *either* to enhance your health *or* to undermine your health.
- When you know you've got choices, then – *and only then* – you can start to make choices.
- When you don't eat something you fancy, that's still a choice you're making. The difficulty is you won't feel like you're choosing if this concept is very new to you. It takes time, thought and repetition before it begins to feel real.

it's easy to assimilate it into your own thinking. When this happens it's as if you are being given orders to follow, as if someone else is in control of you – and you will react to that.

Making threats to yourself – 'you'd better not eat that' or 'don't you dare' – will have the same effect. This language imitates your gaoler who gives you commands, with threats if they aren't obeyed. So you end up feeling like you have no choice but to obey. Even if you know it's you who's doing the commanding, you'll still react as if you are being told what to do.

Feeling Deprived – 'I miss my biscuits.'

If you deny choice you will feel deprived, which is a feeling of self-pity mixed with resentment. If you're more of a rebel, you'll tend to feel angry, irritable, more hungry and even obsessed with food. Feelings of deprivation can lead to apathy and depression and can create symptoms of stress. (1)

Whenever you feel deprived there is sure to be some prohibitive thinking: rules, restrictions and/or threats. *When you change the way you are thinking by reminding yourself of your own choices, these feelings of deprivation will subside.*

Here's an example. For our first few sessions, a client experienced an intense addictive hunger every time she came to see me. When we talked about it, she realised that she had expected me to somehow make her, or order her to, stop overeating. The stirrings of rebellion against this were automatic. After we had established that as far as I was concerned she was free to eat as much as she wanted to, the hunger disappeared.

Treats and Rewards – 'I deserve it.'

Everybody knows forbidden fruits are the sweetest – but usually it's not fruit that gets forbidden but fat, salt, sugar and processed food. If you think of any particular food as forbidden, you'll feel deprived whenever you don't eat it, as if you're being punished. So eating it will feel like a freedom and a reward.

In one study, people in a shopping mall were offered biscuits from a jar and asked to rate their taste on a scale from 1 to 10. Although all the biscuits were exactly the same, they scored higher when they were taken from a jar that was almost empty. *They actually tasted better when they were in short supply!* This doesn't mean you should always stock up with plenty of biscuits. It means it will help you a great deal to remember that there is no shortage of biscuits in your world; the scarcity exists only in your prohibitive thinking.

When we think we can't, mustn't or shouldn't have something, we want it all the more. If we could somehow make celery forbidden in our minds we'd think of it as a treat. We do this because we need to know we are free. One of the worst things that can happen to us is to have our freedom taken away, so it's not surprising we don't like it and instinctively rebel against it. It's this deep, instinctive attraction to something unavailable or forbidden that adds so much power to our addictive desire.

The key is free choice – but in fully acknowledging this, it's essential to keep in mind the consequences of your choices, the complete picture of what it is you are actually choosing. Some choices enhance your health; others will be detrimental to it. *Instead of thinking of food as either 'allowed' or 'forbidden', think in terms of choices you make either to enhance your health or to impair it.*

Strong Compulsions to Overeat – 'I couldn't stop myself.'

This could result from a situation where you became particularly upset about your weight. Perhaps some clothes you tried on didn't fit, or your doctor gave you a warning, or somebody made an insensitive remark about how thin and attractive you once were. Your automatic reaction is one of 'I *have to* lose weight!' and 'I *have to* stop eating so much!' You might at first go into a state of compliance and cut back on your addictive eating. Or you might go straight into rebellion. Either way, you set yourself up for some serious, compulsive overeating sooner or later.

Another, extreme, example is eating food that's gone bad. It's mouldy, rotten and maybe already in the rubbish bin, but the overeater who habitually denies choice can feel strongly compelled to eat it, simply because it's so very much 'not allowed'. People who think this way often become stuck in a permanent state of rebellion: 'I'm not allowed to eat *anything*, so I'm going to eat *everything*, just to prove I'm free to do so.'

Many of us do a version of this, eating things mainly because we think of them as forbidden and we want to confirm to ourselves we are free to eat them if we want to. We may not be aware that this is our motivation at the time, perhaps explaining it by thinking that we 'just can't resist them'. When I've eaten like that I've often (but not always) thought to myself that I don't really enjoy what I'm eating as much as I thought I would. My desire was more to assert my freedom of choice than for the taste or texture of the food.

Rebellious Reaction to Dietary Advice – 'I don't like vegetables.'

A friend of mine, Ellen, asked me to explain the principles contained in a book I was reading about nutrition. I told her that an example of a meal would be about 6 ounces of lean protein with green vegetables. My friend's instant reaction was 'Well, that just makes me want to eat chocolate!' Another example of this rebellious reaction is my pork pie story earlier in this chapter (see page 78).

I'm not suggesting you take on advice without question, simply that you consider the sense of it for yourself – and watch out for the spontaneous rebellion that occurs whenever you think you might be made to eat less. This often happens when a health professional, such as a doctor or nutritionist, has given some specific recommendations about a particular health issue. This doesn't mean you don't still have choices! This doesn't mean you *have to* follow their advice! What it means is that if you follow the advice your health will probably improve – and if you take the step of acknowledging your own free choice in the matter you are much more likely to do that.

Strong Dislike of Natural Hunger – 'I can't stand being hungry.'

At the beginning of this chapter we looked at what it would feel like if you were locked up in a cell and given just enough food to survive. An entirely appropriate reaction to that situation would be anger and resentment, which you would probably feel more strongly whenever you felt genuinely hungry. So you can see that if you have very negative feelings about natural hunger, it may well be because you are not freely choosing it. I'm not suggesting that you go hungry all day; it's just that many people overeat simply because they fear any possibility that they might feel hungry later.

Justifications – 'A bit of what you fancy does you good.'

If you tend to spend much of your time in that mental cell of deprivation, you will appreciate a few keys to let yourself out every now and then. These keys are your favourite justifications for your overindulgences. They provide you with permission to overeat in a world where permission has been removed.

The more convincing the justification is the better, and in order to be convincing the justification must fit the circumstance. An evening alone, a family gathering or a holiday abroad can all seem equally compelling reasons to overeat. Justifications can also be found in any number of physical or emotional upsets. Perhaps you can see that if you were locked up in that cell you might well conjure up an illness in order to get released. In real life this isn't deliberately chosen. It can be quite automatic and unconscious, taking the form of a stomach upset or headache, and can seem a very sensible reason to eat something. Justifications are tricky because they look perfectly reasonable. A *bit* of what you fancy might do you good – but not if you use that justification every time you feel tempted.

When you remind yourself that you're always free to eat anything you want, you will see that you don't need to justify eating anything at all. You can just do it. It's your choice. Then, at least some of your justifications will loosen their grip. More about this later on.

Passivity – 'I have no willpower.'

Feeling hopeless, resigning yourself to the way things are, wishing someone would come along and solve the problem for you or looking for magic cures are all good indications you are not choosing for yourself.

Looking for a magic pill is not going to help you. It will only serve to discourage you once you find that the instant cure you are looking for doesn't exist. When you take control of your overeating it is the result of the choices you and only you can make, not as a result of some gimmick that supposedly relieves you of that responsibility.

A crucial step in owning choice is accepting that nobody else can or should do this for you. *Not only can nobody else do this for you, but you already possess all the magic you need to get this job done.*

Full of Excuses – 'I would eat less, but I just can't.'

'Why Don't You, Yes But' is the name of one of the games from the book *Games People Play* by Eric Berne (2). Played between two people, one is trying to help while the other skilfully avoids making any choices of their own. It begins with the latter describing a problem they have. For example:

A: I live on my own and I cook such huge amounts, I always eat way too much.

B: Why don't you just make smaller amounts?

A: Well, I love to make minestrone soup for example, and there are so many ingredients I always end up with a great big potful.

B: Why don't you freeze some of it, in separate containers?

A: It doesn't freeze well, it loses its flavour.

B: Why don't you keep it in the refrigerator and have it over a few days?

A: Yes, I try to do that sometimes but I find I eat it all in one evening. When it's there, it's so good I just want to keep eating it until it's finished.

B: Why don't you make minestrone only when you've got people coming over who can share it with you?

A: I just do a main course when I have company, like a pasta dish. I wouldn't want to make minestrone as well – I'd be spending all day in the kitchen!

This game is usually played out with someone else, which is one reason I advise you not to discuss with your family and friends anything you define as a 'problem' you have with eating – you're likely to end up playing the game! If it seems as if someone else is trying to make you do something about your overeating, they might be welcomed initially (compliance) but ultimately resisted and resented (rebellion).

You might find yourself playing 'Why Don't You, Yes But' with me as you read through this book. I may make a suggestion, and you automatically react with a 'yes, but' objection to it. You can easily stop this when it happens by asserting your own choice to do whatever you want to do. Owning choice produces results. If the minestrone-maker really owned her choices she would find her own solution. While she thinks of herself as a victim of circumstance, she'll never make any real progress.

And that's precisely where the magic happens; when we own our problems and recognise that we are the source of the solutions. Especially when it comes to eating, because that can be so completely within our control.

The Last Supper – 'I'd better eat while I still can.'

Many people know they overeat because of a sense that it might be their last chance to do so. Of course it isn't your last chance but that can often be the feeling that drives you. Maybe you overeat on the day before starting a diet, but it's also common to overeat not because you've committed yourself to a diet but because of a permanent, albeit vague idea that *all this overeating is going to have to stop*.

Any time you actually try to make a commitment to eat less, this attitude destroys any sense of free choice. A commitment means making one choice that will last into the future; once you've committed yourself you've said goodbye to your freedom of choice. Instead of *commitments*, by all means form *intentions* – and make your choices as you go. When you keep in mind the very real possibility of overeating in the future – later today or tomorrow perhaps – you will have a far greater ability to eat less in the present time.

Way of Life – 'I don't have the time.'

Avoiding the responsibility of choice is a way of life that extends far beyond eating issues. Especially common are those people who take on an inappropriate amount of responsibility for others. They are obsessive care-takers and rescuers, and their entire lives revolve around trying to sort out other people's problems. *They take responsibility for everyone but themselves*.

Low self-esteem drives this way of life: it's an attempt to gain self-worth by fixing things for others. People who live like this may appear to be saints or martyrs, but they drop out on their responsibilities to themselves, and so lose out on strengthening their true self-esteem.

They may justify their lifestyle by telling themselves 'I would look after myself more, but I'm so preoccupied with looking after him/her/them, I can't possibly cope with it all. If only they sorted their lives out, then I'd be able to sort myself out.'

If you recognise yourself in this, it will be important for you to make changes here too, in order to create a bit of space for yourself. You might start by simply refusing to rescue others, at least sometimes. Allow them to be who they are and to make their own mistakes. By detaching yourself in this way, you will be inviting them to take more responsibility for themselves – which may be exactly what they need to do.

I'm not suggesting you should stop caring about them. In fact, allowing others to take responsibility for themselves could be the most caring thing you can do. Maybe it's a matter of you no longer trying to make other people do what you think they should do. Stop trying to control others, and you will free yourself up to take control of yourself.

If you see yourself in these words, notice if you're reading this book mostly with other people in mind. It's very likely that many things will apply to people you know – but you could be ignoring its relevance to *you* by thinking in terms of what other people need to learn. For example, Susan, an overweight friend of mine who read an early manuscript of this book, did nothing about her own eating, but started to give advice to friends and family about theirs. The advice, need I say, was not appreciated.

By all means let people know about this book if you think they may benefit from reading it, but I strongly advise you to be cautious about what you say.

Willpower – and How to Use Yours

Willpower is quite literally the power of your will, and the most important thing to understand about your will is that it is *free*. Your will is in your power to choose freely what you will and will not do. When you deny your freedom of choice you deny your free will. *And you can't possibly use your will effectively while you deny it.*

This is how you undermine your willpower. When someone says 'I have no willpower' it's the same as saying 'I'm not owning my choices'. One of the most common mistakes is to consider the consequences of a certain course of action and then to conclude that you have no options. So watch out for lines of thinking such as:

▌ 'If I want to lose weight, then *I have to* stop eating so much.'
▌ 'If I want to stay in control of my eating, then *I can't* eat any more ice cream.'
▌ 'If I take control of my eating, then *I won't be able* to eat everything I want.'

This is *false reasoning*. You can want something sincerely, even desperately, but this never removes your free choice in the matter. The only time you wouldn't have completely free choices about your eating decisions is if you were locked up in that cell. You wouldn't be overeating, but it wouldn't be your choice. Whenever you notice this way of thinking, correct it to thoughts such as these:

> *I'm not suggesting you go ahead and eat everything you want!*

- ■ 'Yes, I do want to lose weight, but I could continue to overeat and put on even more.'
- ■ 'I do want to stay in control of my eating, but I still have the option of eating addictively.'
- ■ 'I'm more likely to control my overeating when I acknowledge that I am able to eat anything and everything I want.'

I'm not suggesting you go ahead and eat everything you want! And I'm not suggesting that you make a point of consuming all your favourite 'forbidden fruits'. What I'm saying is, if you remind yourself you can eat anything you want, then you will be able to make a choice. You need to know you have a choice before you can make one. What I'm talking about is a change in attitude. It's simply another way of thinking.

You might resist acknowledging choice because you then blame yourself for choices you've made in the past. Perhaps you feel guilty and think 'It's all my fault'. But blaming yourself is not the same as owning choice; it's judging yourself.

Owning choice means independent thought and independent decision-making. You recognise that you are the one who determines what you do, that your actions are up to you and nobody else.

Which choices are going to support our health and which will undermine it may not always be clear, and sometimes we'll get it wrong. We have so much choice when it comes to food! We are confronted with decisions throughout the day about what to eat and when to eat it, what is good for us and what is harmful, how much of it to eat, and whether or not it really is what we want at that time.

So often, though, we abdicate. We get stuck in our habits or follow what everyone else around us happens to be doing.

So often we simply adopt the choices others have made: our family, our peers, our culture, and especially the food industry. In order to make changes, you'll need to gain some knowledge of the facts, and be willing to challenge some of the assumptions you've been making about what you're eating.

When we started out in life, as infants, we didn't have much of a choice about what we ate. Owning choice is a long process which begins when we first put food into our own mouths. Then we begin to make choices about what we will and will not eat, and eventually learn to shop and cook for ourselves or go out to restaurants and order our own meals.

As infants we demanded instant gratification; the ability to delay gratification is something we can develop as we mature. Owning choice is about examining and weighing up instant versus delayed gratification.

Addictive overeating, of course, is very much about instant gratification. In eating less, your gratification could be delayed by hours, days – or even by decades! For example, you could choose not to overeat in the evening for the gratification of a good sleep that night. Or you could choose not to snack on chocolate for the gratification of having more energy during the day. And you could even be choosing fresh, green vegetables instead of takeaways for the extremely delayed gratification of a fit and healthy old age. (3)

Owning choice isn't a decision you make once and that's it. It's not a permanent state. But when you develop the habit of re-creating it over and over, it becomes easier and more natural with practice. The point is to begin. It takes some time and effort, but you will start to feel better immediately.

You'll know when you're doing it because you will be able to make changes in your eating and feel good about those changes. You'll feel more powerful and more hopeful that you've got something which will last.

You'll know when you're doing it because you won't feel deprived when you choose not to eat something – even though you fancy it! This is so important in taking control of addiction. It's practically impossible to stay motivated if it feels as if you are depriving yourself.

You'll know when you're owning choice because you'll experience less guilt and higher self-esteem. This is one reason why self-esteem is a more effective motivation than losing weight. You may lose weight while you are 'locked up' in a diet, but if you are not owning your choices, your self-esteem doesn't necessarily improve.

No matter what happens, you are going to be thinking about food, on and off, for the rest of your life. You'll have thoughts about food every day, at many times throughout the day. You don't have a choice about that! What you do have a choice about is the quality of those thoughts. If you begin to think in ways that cultivate an unrestricted attitude towards food, the benefit to you will become obvious. This *doesn't* mean that you'll never stop eating – as long as you keep in mind the whole picture of what you're choosing.

This isn't an easy, magic solution, but genuine self-esteem is your reward, and my hope for you is that you discover just how exciting that can be. In the next chapter we'll look more closely at how to go about putting choice into practice.

IN OTHER WORDS: SANDRA

I was anorexic for only a short time before developing a compulsive eating and bingeing problem, which I now recognise as rebelling against prohibiting certain foods in certain amounts.

After several successful years of psychotherapy, I resolved most of the emotional issues I linked with food and eating. But to my disappointment I still suffered from addictive behaviour, including compulsive eating, over-eating, compulsive exercise and eating too little. I believed that discipline was the answer: eat enough, but not too much.

But trying harder was fruitless until I accepted freedom and responsibility. It wasn't more rules I needed. It was the knowledge that I was free to eat when and what I wanted: free to starve myself; free to exercise or not; free to binge. Only when I accepted that I was free to take any of these actions could I take responsibility for my choices.

Now, when I'm presented with a choice about food or exercise, I remind myself that I am free to do anything. Then, I ask myself what I want to do. Sometimes I get it wrong, but fine-tuning is part of living.

Taking Control

- If you often have strong cravings for a certain food, it's probably because you consider it 'illegal', and may have done so for a long time. Tell yourself before, during and after eating such food 'I'm allowed to eat this' and 'I can eat as much of this as I want, any time'. Give yourself permission, over and over again, to eat anything and everything you want – and to continue to do that.

- You might fear giving yourself this freedom because you think you will then go ahead and eat anything and everything you want! And you may actually do some of this to begin with because you may recognise choice only superficially. This can be a long-term, deep-seated attitude, which won't go away in an instant. I do want to encourage you to continue with this, though, because you will only be able to take genuine control of your eating when you think in terms of the free choices you are making.

- Choose the consequences along with the food. For example, 'I choose to eat this packet of biscuits *and* the drop in energy I get after the sugar rush *and* the sense of regret and failure I usually feel after I eat like this.'

- Think: 'I can eat anything I want' every time you consider what you want to eat. When you are in a restaurant, let yourself know you can have anything on the menu. When you are shopping for food, tell yourself you can buy anything in the shop. Remind yourself 'This is my choice' every time you eat, *especially* if you regard it as addictive, unhealthy or fattening.

  It may be true that you can't have everything exactly the way you want it. You can't keep eating everything you want without it affecting your health and self-esteem. But even though you don't have a choice about which consequences will follow, you still have free choices about which actions you take.

- Keep these thoughts as private as possible. As much as you can, don't discuss why you are or are not eating something.

If anybody makes a comment about what you are eating, just don't get involved in a conversation about it.

- Possibly the most powerful denial of choice is created by the belief that you 'have to' lose weight (or 'can't' put on any more), and your attachment to this belief may be so strong that it alone causes your feelings of deprivation.

You may want to lose weight, but this is quite different from not having freedom of choice in the matter. The only time you would have to lose weight (you would have no choice) is if you were locked up in a cell and given very little food. While you believe you have to lose weight, you create a state of mind as if you were locked up and so create overwhelming states of deprivation and rebellion.

If it's difficult for you to believe that you don't have to lose weight, try this written exercise:

Write down as many endings as you can to the sentence: 'I have to lose weight because . . .' leaving one line blank in between each sentence. This identifies the thinking behind your false belief. Then go back over what you have written and in each blank line write the true statement. For example:

I have to lose weight because I can't get into my clothes. (*false*)

I could put on even more weight and go out and buy clothes in larger sizes. (*true*)

I'm not encouraging you to put on weight, I'm encouraging you to see that you have choices, so you won't feel deprived whenever you don't eat something. Then – and only then – you begin to move out of the compliance/rebellion cycle and start to take some real control.

- Some people create feelings of deprivation, not because they believe 'I have to lose weight' but because they believe 'I have to control my eating' or 'I have to eat less' or 'I have to stop overeating'. The 'I have to' and 'I can't' statements create the same problems described above, and the written exercise can be applied in the same way. Simply start your sentence with 'I have to stop overeating because . . .' (or words that fit best for you) and proceed in the same way.

- Write down six endings to: 'If I own my choices about what I eat . . .' Write down whatever comes to your mind: there are no 'right' answers. Here are some endings from clients of mine:

> . . . I won't eat the leftovers from my children's plates.
> . . . I'll eat more vegetables.
> . . . I'll eat less.
> . . . I'll feel a lot better about myself.
> . . . I'll feel more in control of my eating.
> . . . I'll be a lot happier.

I suggest you do this exercise as often as you can; once a day would be good. There are many more similar exercises in Dr Branden's *The Six Pillars of Self Esteem* (see Chapter 4).

Notes

1   Stanford University neuroscientist and stress expert Robert Sapolsky describes a number of experiments that show how stress increases when we have no choice – and even when we just think we have no choice: 'This is an extraordinarily powerful variable in modulating the stress-response . . . the exercise of choice is not critical; rather it is the belief that you have it.' From *Why Zebras Don't Get Ulcers* (WH Freeman, 1994).

2   *Games People Play* (Penguin, 1964) by Eric Berne MD.

3   One long-term study found that children who delayed gratification longer in test situations developed into 'more cognitively and socially competent adolescents, achieving higher scholastic performance and coping better with frustration and stress'. The article ends: 'Postponing gratification sometimes may be an unwise choice, but unless individuals have the competencies necessary to sustain delay when they want to do so, the choice itself is lost.' *Science* (1989) 244: 933–937. And it's never too late to start!

CHAPTER 6

What to Do about Wanting More

When an inner situation is not made conscious, it appears outside as fate.
C. G. JUNG

When we make a choice about anything, it makes sense to know what it is we are choosing. We are going to make much better choices when we understand as much as we can about the alternatives available. When it comes to making choices about an addiction, people often think too simplistically, in terms of: shall I do it or shall I not do it? When we think like this we overlook a crucial factor in our decision-making process. This is our addictive desire.

The addictive desire is the driving force behind any addictive behaviour – and the core challenge in taking control. Whether someone smokes a cigarette, takes cocaine or overeats, what they are doing is satisfying their particular addictive desire. For example, a smoker has an addictive desire to smoke and so they light a cigarette to satisfy it. They satisfy it and they reinforce it at the same time. It's only satisfied temporarily, of course, and before long the smoker will feel another desire, and another cigarette will be smoked. All addictions work the same way: first a desire to do whatever it is you're addicted to, and then doing it, which reinforces the addictive desire, and so on.

As someone who overeats, you have been satisfying and reinforcing your addictive desire to eat, possibly every day for many years. The only other reason there is to eat is a genuine need for nutrition, which is often (but not always!) identified by the natural sign of stomach hunger.

Many people never feel their natural hunger because they feed their addictive hunger before their natural hunger appears. The more extra weight a person carries, the less they eat because of genuine hunger. More often they eat to feed their addiction.

Now we get to the biggest and most common mistake people make when they want to control an addiction: *people usually attempt to take control of addictive behaviour by trying to avoid feeling their addictive desire.* They reason that if they don't feel it, they won't feed it, and so assume they will be in control. Most smokers throw away their cigarettes and avoid the temptations of pubs and friends who smoke. In the same way, those people who overeat in the evenings may keep themselves extra busy – the cinema one night, shopping the next, working late another night – all in a determined effort to keep themselves from feeling an addictive urge to eat.

This kind of strategy, in case you don't already know from experience, is flawed. It's flawed because its success depends on you not having any addictive desire – and that can only be a temporary solution. Even more important, though, it's flawed because it doesn't heal the addiction. Just as with any problem in life, avoiding it doesn't resolve anything in the longer term.

For example, after making a decision to stop eating

chocolate, it could be that you don't have much interest in eating any for a while. You think you're doing well because you're sticking to your intention, but I want to suggest to you that you're not accomplishing as much as you could. As you may well know, as soon as your desire resurfaces and you are lusting after your favourite chocolate treat, you eat it. This is because you never faced your feeling of addictive desire in the first place. Or, you do experience your desire for chocolate, but you see this desire as nothing but negative. Maybe you see it as a sign of your weak will or that your biochemistry is out of balance. Addictive desire is almost always regarded as something to be feared, resented and, if at all possible, eliminated.

Unless you begin to respond to your addictive desire in a more positive way, it doesn't matter how well-intentioned or motivated you are or how long you have abstained. It may look for periods of time like you're in control, but all that's happening is you just aren't having a strong enough feeling of desire or maybe no desire at all. Or you feel it but you're fighting it, so it's only a matter of time before you give in to it.

Whether you're making a resolution not to eat chocolate, going on a diet or cutting out fried foods, *the familiar scenario is to start but not to continue.* You might explain this by thinking it's because you don't have any willpower or that you're incapable of discipline. Another way to explain it is that your addictive desire was initially avoided, and when it could no longer be avoided, you satisfied it.

The big question is: are you willing, ever, under any circumstances, to face your addictive desire to eat? As far as taking control of an addiction goes, the addictive desire is where it all takes place. It's only when you come to terms with your addictive desire that things will really start to change. This way may not be so easy to begin with, but the rewards are both profound and lasting.

Bringing Shades of Grey into Focus

The first step in dealing with your addictive desire to eat is to identify it. What distinguishes overeating from most other addictions is its ability to be fairly invisible, completely confused with necessary eating. After all, someone trying to stop smoking can at least be sure what it is they are trying to stop doing. Any overeater knows that food is as addictive as a drug, but they will obviously eat throughout their lives and can only guess at where their addiction begins and ends.

I'd like to suggest a definition of an addictive desire to eat as a desire for any food you don't really need. But I will follow that up right away by saying that our aim is not to eliminate addictive eating entirely – just to do less of it. Our goal is first to know as much as we can when we may be about to eat food we don't need, and then to develop the ability to do it less and less often.

Addictive desire has two aspects. One is about quantity: it's wanting more food than you need, whether it's healthy or not. The other is about quality: it's wanting things you don't need at all because of their poor nutritional content, and even anti-nutritional content – 'food' you would be much better off without.

As we saw in Chapter 1, it's impossible to define addictive eating precisely. This doesn't mean it doesn't exist or that it can't be recognised and managed. In fact, it's impossible to say *precisely* where a great many things begin and end – a mountain, the dawn or your ankle, to name just a few examples. Nobody can say at which exact point your leg becomes your ankle and your ankle becomes your foot. This doesn't mean you don't have an ankle, that you can't use it or point to it and say 'That's my ankle'!

In the same way, we can say that non-addictive eating, pleasurable as it is and should be, is the food we eat in order to stay alive and in good health. Addictive eating can be eating more than you need at meals, in snacks between meals or both. It's addictive if it's more than you need. Extra weight is a good clue which tells you that's what you've been doing, but it's not inevitable; it's possible to stay slim eating addictive 'food' that does nothing but damage your health.

The problem with addiction, though, is that it's out to deceive you, because that's what an addiction does. Your addictive thinking will have you convinced your leg goes all the way to your toes if that will justify eating another slice of cake! What we need to do is find some way to become more sure. At least to begin with, it can help to use some kind of structure with boundaries that will be tougher to dispute.

The solution is contained in two very simple tools, called Times and Plans. First of all, I'll explain what I mean by these terms, then we'll take a look at how to use them to get more control of your addictive overeating.

Times

Times make it easier for you to identify your addictive desire between meals. This tool helps you to cut down on grazing, picking and snacking between meals, assuming this is what you want to achieve.

This is how you use this tool. Whenever you finish eating, whether it's a meal or a snack, set a Time for yourself. Your goal is to get to that Time without eating anything. To begin with, I suggest you set a Time at least one hour ahead and no more than four hours ahead.

For example, if you finish your lunch at 1.30pm, you might set a Time of 4.30pm. What you have done is made a goal not to eat anything at all until 4.30pm. Then, when 4.30 comes, you don't have to eat at your Time. You might decide to eat something, and when you've finished set another Time. Or you might set another Time without having eaten anything.

By setting Times you will be able to gain a real sense of control over your eating. It may be difficult to know whether or not you are about to eat more than your body really needs but you can be absolutely sure of whether or not it's 4.30!

Plans

Plans make it easier for you to identify your addictive desire at the end of meals. This tool will help you to eat less at meals, if you eat meals that are too large or you continue to snack after your meal is finished.

This is how you use this tool. Just before you start eating, preferably before you take the first bite, you decide what you intend to eat at that meal or snack. You decide how many portions, what size portions, how many courses, how many second helpings you plan to eat at that meal.

You don't need to weigh food or measure it too exactly, and you don't need to have it all in front of you to start with. The idea is to create, just before you begin to eat, a mental picture of what it's all going to be, as accurately as you can judge. You might have decided what to eat days earlier when shopping for the week; the idea is to make the Plan in detail *at the point when you start the meal.*

The point at which you take control of an addiction is when you are experiencing your addictive desire – at those very moments you want to eat addictively.

You always have complete control over choosing what your Times and Plans will be. They enable you to eat less; if you have no intention of eating less there's no point in using them. You'll get the best from them if you present yourself with a challenge. Times and Plans give you the ability to begin to see your addictive appetite more clearly – and it's only when you see it that you can get to work on overcoming it.

The point is that sooner or later you'll want to eat something before you get to your Time. And it's inevitable, when you get to the end of your Plan, you'll want to continue to eat more. This is your addictive desire to eat. And believe it or not, this desire is your golden opportunity to make real and lasting changes in your relationship with food.

The point at which you take control of an addiction is when you are experiencing your addictive desire – at those very moments you want ot eat addictively. In that experience of desire you have a chance to open a door and walk through, and when you do you'll find that things really start to change. You'll be stepping out of your 'comfort zone', but you'll be gaining the ability to be in control of your addictive eating. Real control.

I know this may sound unrealistic at first. I know that I'm

suggesting something unusual, and it's understandable if you're doubtful and hesitant to start with. Just keep an open mind, and let's take a look at this addictive desire to eat and see what we can do about it.

Working through Addictive Desire

Understand It

Your addictive desire is often a thought that pops into your mind and says *let's eat!* Sometimes there can be a sense of urgency to it, as if it has to be acted on immediately. But it can also start as a very ordinary kind of thought which only gets satisfied hours later, after you've gone to the shops, perhaps, or when you've arrived home.

It happens because you get reminded by various things – places, people, thoughts, moods, times of day, days of the week, routines, physical states – which you have associated with eating in the past. It's coming from your memory, but it's a special kind of memory that activates reward pathways in the brain – which is why it's felt as a *desire* or *appetite* rather than as a simple recollection. And this is why it tends to be more strongly attached to addictive kinds of food, especially sugar, wheat, potatoes, bad fats and salt.

Often a particular cue will trigger a desire to eat a specific item. For example, years ago I got into the habit of buying a particular chocolate bar every time I got on a train, so turning up at a station would automatically trigger a desire for one, even though I would never think of them any other time.

Most people can see this sort of pattern to their addictive

eating: what they tend to eat when they're alone at home, when they're upset or bored, when it's four o'clock, when they go to the cinema. This eating has nothing to do with nutritional needs and everything to do with the conditioned response of addictive desire, which is at the heart of all addictive behaviour.

Identify It

Your addictive desire to eat can come in a wide variety of shapes and sizes. Sometimes it can be so subtle you don't even notice it. It can simply be the attraction you feel towards certain items in a supermarket. It can be a brief, reasonable, everyday sort of thought flickering through your mind, which suggests you eat something. If some food is on its way into your mouth, it's possible you are experiencing – and about to satisfy and reinforce – your addictive desire to eat. Becoming aware of this is the first step to taking control.

At other times, though, your addictive desire will feel stronger, like a void that demands to be filled. You'll feel it as a physical sensation in your body which will be quite uncomfortable if it's not satisfied. It may well feel like hunger, and it can be difficult to be sure whether or not it's a genuine need for food.

By using Times and Plans you begin to learn how to identify your addictive desire – *but if you've been overeating for many years this can take some time*. Start out by making your best guess: if it's before your Time or more than your Plan, there's a good chance it's your addictive appetite. And if it's a desire for sugar, for example, you know it's addictive because you don't need it at all in order to stay in good health.

THE ADDICTIVE DESIRE TO EAT

The scientist Pavlov found that dogs could be trained to expect food. They salivated whenever a bell rang, simply because the bell rang when they had been fed in the past. Here is a list of things that, by association, may trigger your desire to eat, simply because you ate in response to them in the past.

Consider how often you have reinforced this connection. This is not to make you feel guilty; it's so you can accept the fact that this brain connection won't magically disappear. It fades in time, when you no longer reinforce it, provided you are choosing to accept feeling it.

Places – *shops, restaurants, your kitchen, your car, the cinema, the pub, your workplace, your parents' home, arriving home*

Circumstances – *cooking, family gatherings, being offered food, travelling, watching TV*

Time of day – *mid-morning, 1 o'clock, mid-afternoon, time to go to bed, noticing you haven't eaten anything for a while*

Your senses – *sight, smell and taste of food, advertising and product packaging*

'Negative' emotions – *boredom, sadness, grief, frustration, anger, self-pity, fear, anxiety, stress, self-blame, embarrassment, regret, loneliness, rejection*

'Positive' emotions – *enjoyment, happiness, celebration, relaxation, accomplishment, feelings of connection and intimacy*

➤

Physical sensations – *aches and pains, changes in menstrual cycle, symptoms of stress, feeling tired, drop in blood sugar, noticing your stomach isn't full*
Altered states of consciousness – *being drunk or under the influence of 'recreational' drugs*

• *These associations are often made unconsciously, so you might not be aware of the cue or of your addictive desire to eat. You just find yourself eating again. Times and Plans will help you gain awareness of your addictive desire to eat. It's not essential to identify each cue.*
• *You could experience two or more of these cues simultaneously, and even natural hunger as well. Use the tools of Times and Plans to determine when and how much to eat.*
• *Remember, it's your choice: either satisfy and reinforce your addictive desire, or accept the uncomfortable feeling of wanting to eat in return for some specific improvement in the quality of your life.*

Choose It

Any time you allow yourself to feel your addictive desire, it makes a *huge* difference to remember that you are *choosing* to feel it. You don't *have to* feel it because you could satisfy it. It's your choice. If you forget that you have choices, the addictive desire becomes exaggerated, and it can become exaggerated in different ways:

▉ it can become more frequent, so you want to eat more often

- it can become more intense, turning into a strong feeling of craving
- it can last longer, as a persistent nagging or obsession

For example, you might feel an intense addictive desire as soon as you set a Time because you're assuming you *can't* eat anything until you get to that Time. You may even resist setting Times in the first place because it feels like you're putting yourself into the no-choice cell of deprivation.

It is draining to try to control your eating while you are in a mental state of deprivation, so keep reminding yourself that you always have choices about whether or not you satisfy the desire. If you remember that, you will be able to regard Times and Plans as *tools to use* rather than *rules to obey*. Using these tools will help you gain a better grasp of choice.

If you still don't fully understand this distinction, reread Chapter 5, working on the exercises at the end. If the concept of choice is new to you, it may take a while for it to become real. This doesn't mean it won't work eventually. It just means you need to be persistent. Keep reminding yourself that you can eat anything at any time, and as much as you want. Then, make the genuine, free choices you really do want to live with.

End a Meal with It

Often, just eating an ordinary meal will trigger your addictive desire. This is very common. You might even begin your meal not so interested in eating, but by the end of it your addictive desire is in full swing and you want to go on and on and on. By choosing to feel this desire, you finish your meal still wanting more. You let yourself feel unsatisfied. *This is incredibly powerful, because then you directly confront the addiction.*

When you simply let yourself experience those feelings of desire instead of feeding them, and without getting upset about them, then you are in a very strong position of control. You are able to say 'Yes, that second helping looks wonderful and I know I would enjoy eating it, but I don't have to satisfy this desire for more.' And you'll be able to do that any time, with any food you desire.

> **By working through your addictive desire, you gradually diminish the power of your addiction to food.**

You may not be able to make this change in an instant, but it will help you a great deal to consider going in that direction. Allowing yourself to feel unsatisfied is likely to be the most challenging concept for you to grasp – and by far the most effective when you do.

Value It

The idea is that you freely choose to feel your addictive desire, rather than satisfy it by eating or trying to make it go away by some other means. It is possible to see it as a positive experience – an opportunity. Focus on what you are gaining in self-control and self-esteem, not on what you are losing (a second slice of cake, for example). See it as a trade-off: 'I could eat the cake, but if I accept this feeling of desire I have for the cake I'll gain more control of my eating.'

By working through your addictive desire, you gradually diminish the power of your addiction to food. In fact, *the strength of your addiction could be measured in terms of how much you don't want to feel your addictive desire to eat.* This is what leads you to be out of control in the first place. The addictive desire cannot be permanently avoided, and while you are not prepared to feel it without satisfying it, you are at the mercy of your addiction and its whims. You eat whenever you happen to have a desire to do so, and you'll inevitably continue to overeat.

A binge is an unsuccessful attempt to satisfy an addictive desire. Your attempts to satisfy it keep it going, especially when it's fuelled by a persistent emotion, such as anxiety or loneliness. As it's impossible to satisfy, the desire only abates when you become preoccupied with thoughts of self-loathing and feelings of extreme fullness.

So you can value the uncomfortable feeling of desire because satisfying it is more uncomfortable in its own way. Then you stop trying to satisfy something that is *fundamentally unsatisfiable*.

Face It Directly

A diet/weight-loss way of thinking will lead you to substitute something 'innocent' in an attempt to satisfy your addictive desire. As a result, you end up consuming enormous quantities of things such as sunflower seeds or tea. Or maybe you substitute a pot of low-fat yoghurt for a fatty, sugary dessert at the end of a meal. I once met a weight-loss group leader who would eat four heads of iceberg lettuce at once, with no dressing. Clearly she was feeding an addictive desire for something else.

I don't want to suggest that you never substitute healthy food for junk food because there will be times when that's a very good idea. For example, if you rarely eat fruit it might be good to do so instead of snacking on chocolate in the afternoon. But if this is your strategy for dealing with addictive desire, it won't take you very far. It falls short because you're still not managing the desire directly – and that will be crucial at times.

In order to do that, you deliberately choose between feeding your addictive desire or allowing yourself to feel it. Substituting a healthy option can be a way of compromising on that, which means the fundamental conflict doesn't get resolved.

Resolve the Conflict

You find yourself in a state of conflict when you want two different things at once and you can't have both of them:

1 you want to be in control of your addictive eating *and*
2 you experience your addictive desire to eat

This is the essence of withdrawal from any addiction: a conflict which can feel like a battle. I want to suggest that your failures in the past have been because you avoided this conflict. You won't be able to take real, lasting control until you face that conflict. It's the inevitable difficulty that's required to make real change. Times and Plans help you to see it in the first place (see page 105).

The conflict will diminish in time. Addictive eating reinforces addictive eating, because whenever you feed an addictive desire you strengthen it. When you choose to feel the unsatisfied desire you diminish it. The way to weaken your addiction is to be willing to accept your feelings of addictive desire. Then you resolve the conflict, not by avoiding the desire but by working through it. Then, in time, it fades. (1)

Break the Cues

This process can only be carried out in the same situations in which you overeat. Your addictive desire happens because your brain remembers the connection between overeating and a particular circumstance. For example: walking into your kitchen; finishing a work project; feeling bored; watching TV; feeling angry; driving a long distance. *It's only when you are experiencing these things that the particular connections can begin to break down.*

In order to do this, you need to *pay attention* to the addictive desire when it's happening. In recent years, neuroscientists have demonstrated that focused attention actually causes changes in the brain. You'll need to repeat the process a few times. Remember that you have reinforced this particular memory many times, so it's reasonable to take a while to retrain yourself. But it will help you to remember that by deliberately acknowledging your addictive desire and by making a clear choice to feel it, *you are changing the way your brain works*. More about this in Chapter 10.

Be Willing to Live with It

Even though a great many associations fade and even disappear, it's not possible to eliminate addictive desire totally. This might seem to have happened for days or even weeks at a time, but it's very unlikely to leave you forever.

For some people the addictive desire can disappear for a limited period of time. For example, when people overindulge in a big way, whether it's food, alcohol, cocaine or whatever, the binge is inevitably followed by an initial 'crash' phase with no addictive desire at all. Feelings of guilt and regret will predominate and override any desire for more food. The desire returns in time, of course, when the crash phase has passed.

Many overeaters go through 'binge/fast' cycles in this way. The 'fast' or 'diet' phase of the cycle may seem to be your ideal state because you feel little addictive desire, if any at all. It's likely that you have trained yourself over many years not to feel addictive desire at these times – but it doesn't mean you're in control of your addiction.

Your addictive desire might return when you start to notice that you've lost some weight, that your stomach feels flat or that you are getting into your jeans. It might be when you come across something so tempting and delicious that you break the restrictions you had imposed. Or when you encounter a significant cue for the first time, such as feeling angry. Or it might be simply remembering that you haven't had your favourite, mad binge for a while. Whichever way, the addictive desire comes to the fore again.

Many people find it tough to accept that this addictive desire for excess food isn't ever likely to go away. But if you think it should go, then when it doesn't you'll probably assume it's either a failure on your part or of this method. It does fade, though, and it does become something you can live with very happily. Just remember that it's the presence of the desire, not its absence, that gives you the opportunity to take real control and make real, lasting changes. It's not your enemy, but your friend.

Be Aware of It

A great many overeaters go into a kind of trance when they eat in an addictive way, so that they aren't even aware they are eating, let alone feeding an addictive appetite. This is automatic and (obviously!) unconscious so it's tough to break in one go.

There's no need to despair if this happens to you. You can simply face your addictive desire whenever you start to become aware of what's happening. You still have a choice – even in the middle of a binge or halfway through an enormous meal – to stop eating and start to work through your feeling of addictive desire. For some people that's the place they start to take control.

The more you work with the techniques and ideas in this book, the more you'll get used to the idea of experiencing your unsatisfied addictive desire to eat. You will become more aware of it and it will become more acceptable to you. And as this happens, you'll go into that trance state less and less often. Even when you do, you'll be able to get yourself out of it faster. This can be a gradual process, but the more effort you put into it, the more progress you'll make.

Many people find themselves in that trance state almost every time they eat a meal. The addictive desire kicks in after a bite or two, no matter what kind of food it is. You lose awareness and so you lose control. You can regain control as soon as you become aware of what's happening, probably noticing that you're 'shovelling in' the food much too quickly. It takes some time to retrain yourself, but just put your fork down, sit back and take a breath. You may well feel some resistance to doing this because an addictive desire doesn't want you to stop even for a second. Then, by all means continue whatever you have Planned for that meal (see page 106), maybe stopping again from time to time.

Accept It

Accepting your addictive desire to eat means being willing to feel it, without satisfying it, fighting it, avoiding it or doing things to make it go away. The more you resent it and wish it would go away, the worse it is. The less you resist it, the faster you resolve the conflict it presents. Simply allow yourself to feel it, because it's your resistance to it that makes it more persistent and more intense.

Some people deal with their emotions in the same way. They think positively about having 'negative' feelings, whatever they are. They accept that these difficult emotions are part of life and that to face them and feel them is more beneficial than trying to avoid and ignore them. For similar reasons, it's in your best interest to accept your addictive desire to eat, relaxing as much as you can and letting it be there. (2)

Accept Yourself

Whenever you feel your addictive desire your first reaction may be to blame yourself, perhaps judging yourself as greedy, indulgent or worse. You'll be more accepting of the feeling of desire when you accept yourself for having it. Remember that the only reason you're feeling the desire is because you ate addictively in the past, not because you are fundamentally flawed as a human being. And probably the main reason you ate addictively in the past is because you live in a food-addicted culture. Forgive yourself for the overeating you've done. A sense of humour about it and about yourself will help you a great deal.

Do It for Yourself

Being in a state of desire and conflict is difficult and uncomfortable. If you try to do that *primarily* to improve your appearance you will probably feel deprived, and this is likely to backfire on you. Remember from Chapter 3 that thinking exclusively in terms of wanting to lose weight is a negative kind of motivation. It's your *private* experience of higher self-esteem and improved health and vitality that leaves you feeling like you've gained something when you choose to accept feeling your addictive desire, instead of feeling like you're missing out on something.

Applying Times and Plans

Don't underestimate the value of Times and Plans. The effectiveness of these tools lies in their simplicity. They are flexible from day to day, adaptable to your unique needs and – *most importantly* – self-determined. They are very power-ful tools – but only if you use them in a rigorous way. If you use them half-heartedly, you'll get half-hearted results.

Here are some of the finer details about putting these tools into practice:

■ *Sticking to Times and Plans, but still feeling like you've eaten too much:* It makes sense to set a Time when you think you'll be ready to eat again, but you'll need to learn through trial and error how far apart to set the Times and how much you really do need to Plan at each meal. As you practise, you'll learn what to Plan at each meal so you'll be ready for more food when your next meal is due.

Estimating exactly how much you need to eat will *always* be guesswork. You can do this in a controlled way, though, by using the tools of Times and Plans. Just remember for next time, and know that it's perfectly normal to eat more on some days and less on others. After you have had some experience with this, and on the days when it fits your schedule and your nutritional needs, you might want to make the Times further apart and/or the Plans smaller.

▮ *Drinking:* There's no need to set Times and make Plans for drinking liquids. Be aware, though, if you are trying to satisfy your addictive desire to eat by drinking, whether it's juice, tea, soda, water or alcohol.

▮ *Watching the clock:* If you find yourself frequently checking to see if it's your Time yet, this is your addictive desire. It works a lot better to manage that desire, reminding yourself why you aren't eating, rather than impatiently waiting for your Time. After doing this for a while, your addictive desire will begin to fade, so that you just get on with your life until it's time for your next meal.

▮ *Forgetting to set a Time or setting one and then forgetting what it is:* Set yourself a Time as soon as you realise you don't have one. It's best if it's at least one hour after you last ate, and if it's a somewhat challenging space of time ahead. If you keep forgetting your Times, you could write them down.

▮ *Going past the Time without realising:* Either eat or set a new Time.

■ *You don't know when your food will arrive, so you aren't sure when to set the Time:* For example, you know you'll have a meal when you get home, but you don't know exactly when you'll be home. Or you're at a restaurant or someone else's house for a meal. It's fine to set a Time of, say, 6pm or 'whenever I get home', so long as you then don't start to rearrange your schedule so you arrive home earlier! The same applies to food that's being prepared for you by someone else.

■ *Setting the same Times every day:* It's okay to have some standard Times, such as always eating lunch at 1pm. For many people this is necessary. Even so, it's good to consider your nutritional needs as much as possible, instead of keeping to a routine for the sake of it.

■ *Eating while cooking:* When cooking for yourself, you could include the cooking in your Time and Plan, and eat some while preparing it. It's after your Time and in your Plan, so there's no problem. Otherwise, be aware of whether you're tasting something to see if it's cooked and seasoned properly or swallowing mouthfuls in an addictive way. One of the liberating things about this approach is that you don't have to worry about whether you're eating while standing up, travelling, talking, reading or watching TV.

■ *Starting a meal while you feel strong addictive hunger:* Your addictive desire could continue for some time, especially if it's associated with a persistent mood, and this is another value in using Times and Plans. There will be some days when you feel an addictive desire to eat on and off all day, but if you stick to Times and Plans – because you do need to eat sometimes – you'll know you're in control.

- ▪ *Eating from a buffet or shared bowl:* Make your Plan by selecting what and how much you are going to eat and putting it on your own plate. If you want your Plan to include going back for more, be as clear as you can about what that's going to be before you start eating.
- ▪ *Eating before your Time:* A genuine concern for your health, such as feeling shaky or having a hypoglycaemic attack, is a valid reason to eat before you get to your Time.

I Never Deny Myself!

A client told me this recently with a look in her eyes that said: 'and don't you dare suggest that I should do so!' She was telling me that if she has a strong desire to eat something, she has every intention of satisfying that desire, and she has every right to do so. She *does* have every right to do so, and I'm not going to tell her what choices to make. But she will have to live with the consequences of consistently following that course of action – consequences she was not happy with, which was why she was seeing me in the first place.

At first, allowing yourself to feel an unsatisfied addictive hunger might sound like a fate worse than death. But consider the possibilities. When you accept your addictive desire, instead of thinking it shouldn't be there or trying to make it go away, a lot of things fall into place. To achieve this acceptance, you'll need to struggle through some real conflict. Otherwise you may just be skimming over the surface of the problem.

The biggest mistake people make is trying to find an easier solution. Taking control of addictive behaviour is always difficult. It's not impossible, but it makes sense that it's going to present a challenge that requires some effort. It gets easier when you accept that it *does* require effort. Avoiding that truth makes it worse, because as soon as it gets difficult you are incapable of dealing with it. You set yourself up for failure simply because you are not willing to work through the difficulty.

You can continue to resist and resent the difficulty of controlling your eating. Or you can see that this is an inevitable part of the process and regard the difficulty as the sign that you are beginning to take control. In the words of a reader of one of my books, you can 'Learn to walk the line between desiring and having. Just because you *want* something doesn't mean you have to *have* it.'

There may be days when you feel your addictive desire on and off all day long. The more addictive desire you have, the better, because that's the only time you can practise dealing with your problem. And that's the only time you can work through it and allow it to begin to fade. *The decisions that are the toughest to make enable you to make the most progress.*

All this will take time, so be patient with yourself. If you keep at it, there will come a time when you become much more willing to accept feeling your addictive appetite. Regard every obstacle as an opportunity. For most over-eaters this is a very old problem, and it takes a lot of careful thought to turn around. However, in time, as you continue to use these techniques, your addictive desire will be less and less a problem.

Experience your compulsion to overeat and make your peace with it. It's the sign you are not overeating. It's the sign you are keeping your word to yourself. It's the way you apply the brakes. It means you need no longer be afraid of situations which you associate with addictive eating. You can create, in the words of a client of mine, a relationship with food that is 'a source of contentment and even euphoria, rather than an abiding sorrow'.

As we've already seen, one challenge we face is identifying our addictive desire in the first place. To some extent we will always be guessing, but we can certainly make our best possible guesses as to what we need and what we don't need to eat. The more you eat to meet your nutritional needs and the less to feed your addiction, the more control you will have. The more you know about nutrition and the effect food has on your health, the better your grasp of addictive desire. This information is what we're going to cover in the next chapter.

IN OTHER WORDS: ANNETTE

When I used to diet, I was often able to push the thought of food away. But I knew it would always come back, and it always did. And I was unprepared. Now, when the desire to eat more than I need comes up (and it still comes up!) I take it as an opportunity to discover what it really is that I want.

Now, the desire to eat is no longer the monster that was always lurking in the background. I am able to recognise it, take a look, and try to establish contact. It's still there, but I know it so much better, much better than I ever thought I would. Sometimes we are fighting each other, but I don't feel helpless any more.

When faced with a chocolate cake, I would desire it intensely. It was almost like being in love. At the same time, I knew I shouldn't eat it. So I ate it and felt bad. Now, ➤

I still sometimes eat it, though most often I don't. But now it is no longer the one I love. It's just a chocolate cake.

The way to get through your addiction is not by denying it or trying to avoid it (which you can't anyway) but by experiencing it. This is a very important and exciting process which gave me access to a lot of information about myself, over and above the eating problem.

I can change. I can decide. I can take charge. I eat food, food doesn't eat me. I don't feel guilty about my desire. I feel it but I don't feed it.

Taking Control

- In a nutshell, this is how to manage your addictive desire to eat at the time it's happening:

— THE OUTLINE —

I have an addictive desire to eat
I have the freedom to eat

Either:
I choose to satisfy this addictive desire
and get the consequences (e.g. regret, fatigue)

Or:
I choose to accept my desire to eat in order to gain
the benefits of being in control (e.g. esteem, energy)

- While The Outline is working for you, you don't need to do anything else. I'm a great believer in the advice 'if it ain't broke, don't fix it'. Use all the rest of the information in this book for troubleshooting. If or when this technique breaks down, then you can investigate the cause of the problem.

- There will be many experiences of addictive desire that you could ignore or dismiss very easily. However, if you practise with these easy ones, you'll be much better equipped to cope with the stronger urges when they happen.

- Pay attention to your own experience of addictive desire, rather than trying to fit it into a preconceived picture of what it should be. It can simply be a thought, but if it's also a feeling, *bring your attention to the sensation in your body*, whatever it is.

- One crucial key is your shift of attention away from the *object* of your desire – the food – to focus on your own *experience* – your thoughts and feelings of desire. It should take just a few moments to deal with those thoughts and feelings, and then by all means get on with whatever you are going to do next. This is not to say that the desire will always be gone in just a few moments, but that you will be able to live alongside it.

- Sometimes the desire will evaporate as soon as you direct your attention to it. At other times it may persist. Just remember that it's okay to have that feeling; breathe and *let it be there*.

- By all means use Times and Plans only in those circumstances where you tend to overeat. So, for example, if you are happy with your eating during most of the day and do all your overeating in the evening, just use Times and Plans in the evenings.

- Availability makes any addictive desire stronger, so if you surround yourself with the food you love, you're likely to experience a more persistent desire. Don't drive yourself crazy with this; find a balance. It's fine if there are some things you prefer not to keep at home.

- It's a good idea to manage your addictive desire at the shops, as that's where many choices to eat are made. It's just a matter of time as to when you actually do the eating which satisfies that desire – in the car on the way home or later that evening. Go up to the products and talk to them (privately!). Acknowledge your addictive desire for them and make your choice, remembering the benefits you gain if you choose to leave them there on the shelf. If you feel deprived of them later on that evening, recall that you were the one who made that choice and think about why you made it. And let yourself know that you can return to the shop tomorrow and make a different choice if you want to.

- Notice how you benefit from using Times and Plans and The Outline, and consider making some notes about this for yourself. It's very likely you will take these benefits for granted later on, and it will be helpful to have as much written down as you can – especially those benefits that have nothing to do with weight loss.

- Keep all this to yourself. Make private choices by telling no one of your Times and Plans. If you don't bring the subject up, you won't invite other people's involvement.

    This obviously applies to your day-to-day life, not to group meetings, counselling or therapy sessions you attend in order to talk through these issues. There's a great difference between discussing the *Eating Less* technique with the help of a counsellor or group, and bringing it into daily conversations with family or friends.

NOTES

1. To summarise a substantial amount of research that supports this, Dr G. Alan Marlatt, a leading researcher from the University of Washington, states: '. . . repeated unreinforced exposure to drug-acquisition cues will lead to the extinction of appetitive urges and craving responses'. Reprinted from *Addictive Behaviors* 15, 395–399(1990) with permission from Elsevier.

2. In *The Six Pillars of Self-Esteem*, Nathaniel Branden writes about the value and practice of acceptance:

   'When we fight a block it grows stronger. When we acknowledge, experience and accept it, it begins to melt because its continued existence requires opposition.

   'To "accept" is more than simply to "acknowledge" or "admit". It is to experience, stand in the presence of, contemplate the reality of, absorb into my consciousness. I need to open myself to and fully experience unwanted emotions, not just perfunctorily recognise them.

   'Accepting does not necessarily mean liking, enjoying or condoning. Acceptance of what is, is the precondition of change. And denial of what is leaves me stuck in it.'

CHAPTER 7

What's for Dinner?

No trumpets sound when the important decisions of our life are
made. Destiny is made known silently.
AGNES DE MILLE, HOLLYWOOD CHOREOGRAPHER

How do you decide what to eat? Do you go for whatever
seems the most enjoyable? If so, how can you know
whether or not your addiction is dictating what you're
choosing?

It's often claimed that there's an instinctive, natural
mechanism that tells us what we need or don't need to eat,
but I have very little confidence in that idea. I'm not saying
some degree of intuition doesn't exist, nor that it is lost
forever for everyone, but it is strongly influenced by
addiction to food. If it were only up to me, I don't think I'd
know which foods were damaging my body until it was too
late. After all, my body couldn't have evolved with an ability
to keep me away from sugar, for example, because even
though it does nothing but damage my health, it's a
relatively recent invention. This is why I prefer to rely on the
advice of others.

Fortunately, I do have this information, and so do you.
We know that people get ill and even die prematurely as a

direct result of eating too much of certain kinds of food and not enough of other kinds. It happens gradually, but it happens, and it continues to happen to an enormous number of people. It's likely that some of the information we are given about nutrition at any time is incorrect, but the approach that rewards us with the best possible health and self-esteem is to eat according to our best evaluation of the advice that's currently available.

There is always going to be controversy in the field of nutrition; no two experts will agree on every detail of the best possible diet. But to me, it is precisely this controversy that makes the overwhelming consensus of opinion on some things so compelling. There really is a great deal of agreement on the harmful effects of refined sugar and wheat, salt and the bad fats – and on the beneficial effects of more natural foods, especially vegetables. (1)

It will help you to read this chapter with the previous six chapters in mind, noticing the impact this information has on your attitude towards:

■ **Motivation** This chapter will help you to develop motivation that strengthens genuine self-esteem and wellbeing, so that if you do need to lose some weight, you'll do it in a way that lasts.

■ **Choice** Own your choices by remembering that nobody is making you do anything against your will. You are free to eat anything you want, in whatever quantities you want, and you never have to make any healthy changes, *ever*. Then, think in terms of making choices *either* to support your health and self-esteem *or* to reinforce your addiction to food, which undermines your health and self-esteem.

■ **Addictive desire** Your addictive thinking will be challenged by this chapter because it gives you powerful reasons not to satisfy your addictive desire.

The Basic Recommendations

■ **Vegetables** – between five and ten servings every day, a wide range of different kinds and colours – raw, lightly steamed or stir-fried in olive oil.

■ **Fruit** – three or four servings every day, preferably raw.

■ **Lean protein** – preferably small amounts at every meal. Free-range, organic poultry and eggs are good sources. Eat fish (especially oily fish such as mackerel, salmon, herring and tuna) twice a week and red meat no more than about once a week. Soya products, pulses, seeds and nuts are also sources of protein.

■ **Starchy carbohydrates** – good-quality brown rice, millet, small red-skinned potatoes, yams and sweet potatoes are best – no more than two servings every day. Rye is the best for bread. If you are going to eat wheat, make sure it's best quality stone-ground.

■ **Fats** – the best are the essential fatty acids found in seeds and their (cold-pressed) oils and in oily fish. In addition, it's fine to eat the monounsaturated fats found in foods such as olives, avocados and olive oil.

■ **Dairy products** (a bit controversial) – limited amounts of whole, organic milk, butter and plain, live yoghurt are best.

Yes, but Why?

I hope you agree that the above recommendations aren't all that complicated. If you're anything like me, though, you'll want to know why you're following them, and that's going to take some explanation. I know that when I understand why I'm doing something I'm much more likely to keep it up. Otherwise, I'm just mindlessly following instructions – and I'm not very good at doing that!

The short explanation is that when we follow these guidelines we will be eating in a way that slows down our aging process. This is not to deny the reality of aging, but we really can keep our bodies as youthful as possible for as long as possible. For example, if I have a choice between developing diabetes when I'm 60 or when I'm 80, I'd prefer to have 20 years free of that disease. And I do have a choice. Every choice about food that I make throughout my life makes a contribution, however small. (2)

These recommendations will feel overwhelming if you are going to try to be a perfectionist about them. There's really no need to do it 100 per cent, though. It's all a matter of balance and degree. If, in the past, you have been able to eat in a healthy way only if you do it 'perfectly', you will find help in Chapter 12.

Here are some basic principles about the effect food has on our bodies which explain how to gain a healthier balance:

Lose Fat, Gain Lean Mass

Bring to mind the image of a pork chop and you have a picture of what we're talking about here. The lean meat is the part of our body we are supposed to have. The fat is what you actually want to lose when you say you want to lose weight.

Unfortunately, a great many people don't understand this distinction and regard *any weight loss at all* as good news. Often, though, they lose lean mass (mostly muscle tissue) and in doing so they have accelerated the physical aging of their body. Some loss of lean mass

It's fairly easy to lose lean mass; losing fat is a much slower process.

might be inevitable as we age, but by speeding up that process we create earlier problems with blood glucose tolerance (insulin resistance), blood pressure, aerobic capacity, bad cholesterol, bone density and the ability to regulate body temperature.

Not only that but your metabolic rate is also affected, because the more lean mass you have, the more calories you burn, even when you're at rest. One pound of lean mass burns between 30 to 50 calories a day while one pound of fat burns less than two. So, the more lean mass you have, the more you'll burn off calories and excess fat.

Most men can lose fat more easily than women as they tend to have more lean mass to start with. And for many people it's much easier to gain fat later on in life because a greater proportion of lean mass has been lost. Even when you're young, though, the more you diet, the more you tend to lose lean mass. And even without dieting as such, poor nutrition and inactivity over a period of time will result in more lost lean mass and a greater tendency to gain fat.

It's fairly easy to lose lean mass; losing fat is a much slower process. Most people who go on quick weight-loss diets, liquid diets and those who use appetite suppressants are losing lean mass weight. Lean mass weighs considerably more than fat (think of that pork chop) so the drop in scale weight can seem encouraging.

You can build and maintain lean mass, so all this is largely reversible. How much lean mass you have is the single most important factor in determining the biological age of your body, so in doing this *you actually make yourself younger*.

Lean mass is supposed to make up about half of your weight, so its relevance is considerable. In building lean mass, exercise is crucial – *but you cannot regenerate body tissues without adequate nutrition*. Our bodies need the basic building blocks (the right kinds of protein, fats and carbohydrates) in order to build and repair the lean tissue – work that goes on every night while we sleep. When you don't eat enough of these essential building blocks (by eliminating carbs, for example, on the Atkins Diet) you are in danger of losing some amount of lean mass. (3)

As muscle weighs more than fat, it's better not to rely on ordinary scales. If you want to find out if you are carrying an unhealthy amount of *fat*, use a measuring system that reads your body-fat percentage. Only then can you accurately gauge your weight in terms of health. A simple guide would be to measure your waistline as scientists now believe it is a very good indicator of health. (4)

Counting calories is too simplistic because it depends so much on what food those calories come from. If the calories come from lean protein and good fats, much of it will not be stored as fat but used to maintain your lean mass, make hormones and repair cell membranes.

The message is to eat in a way that builds and maintains lean mass. You'll lose the fat, keep it off and you'll stay healthy too. And it's never too late to start. (5)

Blood Glucose Balance

So much has been written about this, I would be surprised if you don't already know about this aspect of nutrition. To summarise, whenever we eat any carbohydrates, our glucose and insulin levels rise and fall. Some kinds of carbohydrates cause glucose and insulin to rise and fall rapidly and other kinds more gradually. Different foods have been graded according to this response in what's known as the Glycaemic Index. The kinds of carbohydrate that cause a larger rise and fall in blood sugar levels are rated high on the Glycaemic Index. The carbohydrates that cause insulin to be released more slowly are low on the Glycaemic Index.

However, an improved version of the Index has now been developed and is known as the Glycaemic Load (GL). This adjusts the items in the more familiar Index by taking into account the amount of carbohydrate calories in terms of the volume of the food. So, for example, bananas and carrots are high on the Glycaemic Index but rated much lower in terms of Load. (6)

There is now a great deal of evidence that indicates that high-Glycaemic Load carbs are not at all good for our health. Eating too many of them is associated with fatigue, chronic low blood sugar (mood swings, headaches and dizziness), high triglycerides, lower levels of good (HDL) cholesterol, high blood pressure, the release of cortisol and adrenaline (which makes us feel stressed), late-onset diabetes and heart disease.

And many nutritionists and doctors are now saying that it's the high-GL carbs that are keeping us fat. It seems that when insulin levels are too high our cells create more body fat. (This makes sense when you consider that during World War II, underweight soldiers suffering battle fatigue were given insulin injections in hospital to make them gain weight. It worked extremely well, except that sometimes it induced a coma, so the practice was stopped.)

The challenge for us is that the high-GL carbs tend to be the most addictive: sugar, potatoes and processed grains, including most commercial breads, cereals, crackers, cakes and biscuits. Our bodies respond to all of these as sugars and are not designed to deal with them.

The message is to eat the high-GL carbs less often and, when you do eat them, to balance them with proteins, good fats and low-GL carbs with fibre to slow down the release of insulin. (7)

HIGH-GL CARBOHYDRATES

By far the best sources of carbohydrates to eat regularly are those with a lower Glycaemic Load such as most vegetables, fruits, whole grains, beans and pulses. They are naturally rich in fibre, which slows down the release of glucose.

Here is a list of common carbohydrates with a higher Glycaemic Load, rating 20 or more. They are more addictive, often overeaten, have lower nutritional content and in many cases contribute to over-acidity.

This is not *a list of foods you 'must not' eat, but if you are going to choose to eat less of anything, this is one place to start.*

Grain-based Foods
* *most breakfast cereals, quick-cooking oats or rice,* ➤

puffed rice, puffed wheat
- *white flour and products made from it, white and brown bread*
- *white rice, risotto rice, sushi, couscous*
- *corn, rice or durum wheat pasta, instant noodles*
- *taco shells, pitta bread, bagels, baguettes*
- *pastry, croissants, muffins, waffles and pancakes*

Potatoes
- *baked, mashed, roasted, instant mash, chips/French fries*

Sweeteners
- *table sugar, glucose, maltose, syrups, condensed milk*
- *products containing sugar, such as yoghurts and jams*

Snacks and Drinks
- *rice cakes, crisps and crisp-type products, corn chips*
- *biscuits, cakes, chocolate bars, most fruit and cereal bars*
- *dates, sultanas*
- *shop-bought fruit juices, most sodas, alcoholic beverages*

From 'The Revised International Table of Glycemic Index and Glycemic Load', *American Journal of Clinical Nutrition*, July 2002.

pH Balance

Everything we eat and drink affects the pH of every cell in our bodies, making them either more acidic or more alkaline. Most people are eating food that makes them too acidic, so our bodies continually suffer, and work to restore a healthy, more alkaline, balance.

Over-acidity causes inefficient digestion and poor elimination of toxins, which means poor nutrient absorption, less oxygen and higher toxicity. Symptoms include fatigue, headaches, allergies, skin problems, heartburn, stomach bloating, stomach ulcers, poor concentration, problems sleeping, joint aches and pains.

Over-acidity lies at the root of serious illness and disease; people with degenerative diseases such as arthritis, rheumatism and cancer tend to have very high acidity in their tissues and blood. And over-acidity is behind the loss of calcium from bones, resulting in osteoporosis. This is thought to be because calcium is taken from the bones in order to make the body more alkaline, which is of primary importance. Over-acidity also encourages the growth of unfriendly, 'morbid' bacteria, which develops into yeast and fungus.

The message is to consume less of the most common causes of over-acidity – sugar, wheat, processed foods, hard cheeses, alcohol and meat – and to eat more vegetables which make the body alkaline. (8)

Improved Circulation

As you probably know, the circulation of blood around your body is a transport system which delivers oxygen and nutrients to every cell and takes waste products away to be eliminated. Among other things, our blood transports tiny particles of fat, some of which is needed to repair cells and manufacture hormones, but some kinds of fat do nothing but clog the system, just like an accident on a motorway.

When that starts to happen the whole system becomes less efficient. This may show up as high blood pressure and eventually heart disease, but it can also contribute to many other problems because the delivery of nutrients and elimination of toxins is impaired.

The most well-known of the artery-clogging fats is the saturated kind, found in animal meats and products. But there are fats that are considerably worse: the hydrogenated and trans fats found in most manufactured products. These are artificial fats and oils that have been chemically altered in order to improve their shelf-life. They are found in vegetable oils, margarines and all the products made with them. Unfortunately, there is no legal requirement to list trans fats as an ingredient, but unless you have good information otherwise, it's safe to assume it's in snack foods, most manufactured confectionery, ice creams and baked goods (biscuits, bread, crackers, pastries, pies, cakes, croissants, doughnuts, sausage rolls, etc.), commercial sauces and salad dressings, and any food coated in bread-crumbs, fried or baked with oil (crisps, chips/French fries, chicken, pizza, fish, fish fingers). These fats and oils are very damaging. They are *not metabolised* and cause havoc as a foreign, sticky molecule that stays inside our arteries. That's why nutritionists are now recommending we use olive oil and/or butter, and fry seldom, if at all.

Fewer Free Radicals, More Antioxidants

Our health and biological age are also determined by levels of 'free radical damage'. Free radicals are highly charged molecules that are by-products of metabolism, and it is very much to our benefit to keep levels as low as we can. Otherwise, these free radicals go after our DNA, protein and fat, damaging them by stealing electrons. This free radical damage to our own molecules is known as *oxidative stress* and is associated with all the degenerative diseases – heart disease, hardened arteries, high blood pressure, stroke, cancer, arthritis, adult-onset diabetes, Alzheimer's, Parkinson's, cataracts, macular degeneration and depression. At the molecular level, the more oxidative stress to our DNA, proteins and fats, the quicker the onset of one or several of these chronic degenerative diseases. Which disease shows up first may simply be a matter of the weakest link in our own genetic make-up.

The most serious source of free radical damage is smoking, which is why it's so very bad for our health in so many ways. Free radicals also accumulate faster as a result of exposure to environmental pollution, x-rays and sun rays, stress, alcohol, excessive exercise, any drugs and medications, injury and disease. As for food, both the quantity and the quality of what you eat will determine how much free radical damage will occur. Some amount of cell damage is inevitable – just as aging is inevitable – but the damage accumulates, so the older we get the more likely the effects will become serious problems.

We can keep free radical damage to a minimum in three ways:

1 by avoiding damaging the cells as much as possible in the first place
2 by eating foods that neutralise the free radicals
3 by eating less, and more wisely

Free radical damage is neutralised by the antioxidant nutrients found in vegetables, fruits, whole grains, nuts and seeds. However, no other kind of food comes close to vegetables and fruits for antioxidant content.

Every time we eat natural, fresh foods, the antioxidants they contain get rid of significant amounts of free radicals, reducing oxidative stress. The different colours of these foods – reds, yellows, browns and greens – indicate different varieties of antioxidants, which is why it's good to eat a wide variety. The antioxidants do not work in isolation, but together as a team, which is why vitamin pills are not much help. At last count, about 7,500 different antioxidants have been identified, so the few dozen or so in a vitamin supplement don't fit the bill.

The quantity of food you eat will have a direct impact on free radical production as well. The more food your body has to process, the more free radicals get generated. Scientists have shown that the lifespan of every kind of animal – from bacteria to humans – can be extended *by reducing calories while maximising nutrition*. This strategy is perhaps the most powerful one for reducing oxidative stress.

The digestion of *any* food results in some amount of free radical production, so if the food you eat doesn't deliver plenty of antioxidants, *you've created a deficit!* The message is to consume antioxidants daily because some amount of cell damage occurs daily. The immediate benefit is to your immune system, vitality, complexion and mood. (9)

'I Already Eat Healthy Food'

This is something I've heard from many clients. Unfortunately it usually means that someone has already made some changes but closed themselves to making any more.

The way to eat less, and to do that in a way you can maintain long term, is to continue to raise your standards about healthy eating. Expect resistance along the way, though, because *there's still an addiction influencing your choices*.

This means you will experience addictive desire – especially for the high-GL carbs, bad fats and salt. It is possible to eat healthy food in an addictive way (far too much fruit, for example) but most people find their addictive desire is strongest for foods with the more addictive qualities.

If I chose my food influenced *entirely* by my addictive desire, I'd only eat things like pizza, fry-ups, pork pies, pastries, ice cream and chocolate-covered raisins, to name but a few. I suspect that I wouldn't eat fruit or green vegetables at all, and certainly not every day. I'm not alone, of course. Many of my clients tell me that they don't really fancy vegetables, especially not as the main part of their diet. This is all part of the addiction. When you are accustomed to feeding your addictive desire, you won't find nearly as much gratification in food that doesn't contain those more addictive elements. An apple just won't satisfy as much as an apple pie with custard will.

> **The more food your body has to process, the more free radicals get generated.**

Most people settle for a compromise somewhere between their nutritional needs and their addictive pleasures. A nod in the direction of nutrition is used to justify addictive eating again. For example, you'll eat steamed broccoli – but only if it's smothered in cheese. You order a side salad to start with – but just so you can convince yourself that your pizza lunch was a healthy one. You snack on fruit in the afternoon instead of something sugary – so you reward yourself with biscuits later on.

As we saw in Chapter 1, any addiction is pleasure-seeking behaviour. If your taste buds always have the last word, you will continue to eat addictively because they are, at least in part, the expression of your addictive desire.

> *An apple just won't satisfy as much as an apple pie with custard will.*

It could be that you've made healthy changes in your diet to the point at which they come into greater conflict with your addictive desire. You've made some concessions, but continue to justify overeating the high-GL carbs, bad fats and salt in some form. Not only do you not need these because they don't supply you with essential nutrients, but the chances are you eat them in quantities that are actually dangerous to your health. *As far as your health is concerned, you'd be much better off without them.*

Anti-nutrition

A great many people have the idea that they eat what they need, and then overindulge in the naughty, fun foods that unfortunately pile on the pounds. For example, they choose a 'sensible' salad and follow it with a 'treat' of chocolate. The trouble is, as far as your health goes, the 'treat' could be undoing much of the health benefit of the salad. The addictive 'treats' have the effect of cancelling out other nutrients, so they aren't just empty calories; eating them actually contributes to nutritional deficiencies and more oxidative stress.

The chocolate bar contains sugar, of course, which provides no nutrition whatsoever and robs the body of essential nutrients, especially chromium and B vitamins. And, as we've already seen, it makes the body more acidic and upsets the blood glucose balance. As well as sugar, most commercial chocolate bars are filled with hydrogenated and/or trans fats which, among other things, block the absorption of essential fats as well as clogging arteries.

Most, if not all, manufactured 'food' is, in fact, anti-nutrition and not food at all. We are surrounded by it. It's more addictive, which means we are likely to be more attracted to it than real food. A good rule of thumb is: if it's packaged, marketed and advertised, it's very likely to be addictive anti-nutrition. Advertising costs a great deal of money, which means someone expects to make lots of money as a result, and, as any drug dealer knows, addictive substances are by far the easiest things to sell. This is why there's highly addictive, high-GL carbs, fat and/or salt in almost all commercially prepared foods, and this is why people keep eating them.

People who design and produce 'food' (i.e. things to eat) are guided by what will sell – *not by a concern for your well-being*. They care as little about your health as do the people in the tobacco industry, which I don't find hard to believe, given that the same company owns Marlboro cigarettes, Nabisco and Kraft Foods. (10)

What assists their marketing is that so many people assume they are healthy because they are not hospitalised or don't have obvious signs of pain and physical deterioration. This comes from having a standard of health based on more dramatic symptoms of illness. But just because you don't have a serious illness, this doesn't mean you are in the best possible state of health. A serious illness is usually the final sign of a long-established state of ill health.

You can change your standard of health by paying

attention to more subtle symptoms and finding out how the food you eat affects them. Do you feel tired during the day? Do you suffer from indigestion? Do you get headaches or PMS? Are you susceptible to infections, colds and flu? *These, and many more, could be early warning signs that you are eating addictively much too often: too much in quantity and too little in quality.*

I do want to lodge a protest here and state that I don't particularly like this state of affairs! I know this sounds like my addiction talking, but I would much prefer that pepperoni pizza was as good for my health as cabbage. I'd rather eat fish and chips than salad for lunch and I'd rather have crisps than pumpkin seeds for snacks.

Unfortunately, it doesn't matter what I want. My body just isn't designed to work that way. It's like wanting to run my car on tap water instead of expensive petrol: it doesn't matter how much I want it or how much I complain about it – *it just doesn't work!*

Whenever I fight against reality, it's me who gets the bruises. The more I fight it, the more bruised I get. The bruises in my case were acid indigestion, a substantial loss of energy and a very real dent in my self-esteem that I became aware of only when I started to make changes. The more wisely I eat, the better I feel – physically, mentally and emotionally. That's just how it is. You don't have to take my word for it. Just check it out for yourself.

You will need to take great care, though. The culture we live in tends to regard addictive food as normal, wholesome and even something to be highly prized. You will need to outwit not only the food industry, but also the slimming industry, possibly your family and friends and, most of all, your own addiction to food.

Increase Quality, Decrease Quantity

It's no coincidence that we tend to overeat those foods that are the most damaging to our health. These foods trigger chemicals in our bodies which, although they are not good for us, make us feel good. To make matters worse, if we think we aren't allowed to eat these foods, we'll just want them all the more and rebel by eating them whenever we can find a good enough excuse.

There's no other reason for these products to exist. A kind of collective denial in our culture makes them seem acceptable, but apart from satisfying our addictive desire, all those products do is make us ill. Addiction is the only reason they're eaten, the only reason they're bought, and the only reason they're made in the first place. (11)

This is important to see because making changes in what you eat could be as significant, if not even more so, as making changes in how much you eat. Remember that you always have the freedom to eat anti-nutritious foods. Just because they're bad for you doesn't mean they are forbidden. It just means that eating too many of them will make you ill – if they're not already doing so. Remember that by managing your addictive desire for them you gain in health and vitality. *There is also great pleasure to be found in good health, self-control and stronger self-esteem.*

When we eat as nature intended, both in terms of the quality and quantity of food, we will look, feel and be our best. Even though what nature intends may not always be clear, a sincere effort in that direction will bring us far more rewards in terms of health and self-esteem than deciding it's all too confusing to bother with.

The more you develop the skill of managing your

addictive desire to eat, the easier this process will become. There's no need to eliminate your addictive eating completely. Simply aim to do it less often. The truth is that there are 'good' foods and 'bad' foods in that there are foods that enhance your health and foods that

> *Just because they're bad for you doesn't mean they are forbidden.*

undermine it. Make health your priority and you have the best possible motivation when managing addictive desire.

IN OTHER WORDS: CARRIE

I have always struggled with a tendency to 'comfort eat' in times of stress. Comfort eating for me means reaching for foods which are high in sugar, particularly chocolate, and eating them in large quantities to satisfy an emotional need I can't always put a name to. In my 20s I started to look for solutions.

I became interested in some books that took the approach that all food is just food. In our minds we should make no differentiation between 'good' foods and 'bad' foods, and we should preferably surround ourselves with copious amounts, by way of soothing ourselves. In addition, we should continually try to analyse our emotional reasons for comfort eating in an effort to use that self-examination as a distraction from eating when not hungry or from eating too much.

I tried to follow this advice for many years, but it never seemed to work. If I surrounded myself with sugar and chocolate, I only ate it, and my pattern of comfort eating continued unabated. ➤

When I discovered Gillian's book, I felt excited on reading it. It made a refreshing change from what I'd read before, and at last I felt I could really relate to what was being said. I found the answers I'd been looking for to get my chaotic eating under control.

The answer was not to indulge my emotional justifications for comfort eating. Nor was it to surround myself with high-GI comfort foods with the intention of persuading myself they were just another harmless food source. The fact that I knew I could still choose was important, to quell my rebellious approach to eating. My motivations were to get in control of my eating, even though everything else in my life might be chaotic, and to reduce stress.

The key messages of Gillian's book that have helped me are: to regard overeating as an addiction which need not be indulged; to avoid buying in copious amounts of 'comfort foods' which merely create temptation rather than familiarisation; and to understand that all food cannot be regarded as harmless. These messages are all contrary to what other writers have said and at last I understand why their methods didn't work.

Having experienced a good deal of stress in my years as a single parent, it was crucial for me to understand the link between high-GI foods and the release of cortisol. I rarely choose these foods now. Instead, I choose nutrient-rich foods, including a lot of vegetables and fruit, to combat stress.

Having absorbed Gillian's messages, something amazing happened. After 25 years of struggling with chaotic eating, I now have the control and enjoyment around food that I have yearned for.

Taking Control

- As much as you can, notice whether you are eating to satisfy your nutritional needs or your addictive desire. Tell the truth to yourself whenever you are about to eat something that's anti-nutritious. You'll want to eat it; you'll be free to eat it; you'll try to justify eating it – and, at least sometimes, you probably will eat it. Just get into the habit of identifying it for what it is and don't try to kid yourself that it's real food.

- Broadly speaking, there are two distinct styles of addictive eating:

  1 eating a complete and balanced diet, and then more than you need, either in quantity or quality or both

  2 eating poor-quality food without any serious attempt to meet nutritional needs

  If you identify with the first style, use Times, Plans and The Outline to eat less of what you don't need (see pages 105–28). Addictive thinking is behind the second style, too. Use the techniques to manage your addictive desire for 'convenience' (sugary, fried, refined and processed) foods. Remember that fresh, green vegetables might not satisfy your addictive desire – but that's no reason not to eat them!

- You may need to put some effort into discovering where to get good food daily. Actively seek out the recipes, shops and restaurants that will give you access to better-quality food. Once you've created these new habits, they will last you a lifetime.

- If you don't read labels you'll have no idea what you're eating! However, be aware that labels on food products are often designed to deceive you. As just one example, ingredients must be listed in order of amounts used in the product, with the main ingredient first. But contents can be divided into two listings (two different kinds of sugar, perhaps) so it appears to contain smaller amounts. What's best is to eat food that's so natural it doesn't need a label in the first place.

- Calorie content alone isn't a complete guide to what's best to eat because high-calorie foods can provide you with important nutrients. Nuts, for example, are high in iron, essential fatty acids and vitamin E – and they don't have to be coated in addictive oil and salt! Beans and lentils are good sources of minerals, fibre and B vitamins. Avocados make your body more alkaline and are full of healthy mono-unsaturated fat.

- There's often confusion around chocolate because the cocoa itself is rich in healthy antioxidants and flavanols, while most chocolate products are largely composed of unhealthy sugar, wheat and bad fats. You can buy 100 per cent cocoa powder in supermarkets and concoct your own chocolate treats, preferably with a sweetener that does not upset blood sugar levels, such as stevia. (See my website, www.eatingless.com, if you don't know about this product.)

- The term 'refined' in describing sugar and flour is extremely misleading. The 'refining' process was developed for commercial reasons in order to prolong the shelf-life of food: these products have been 'killed' so they won't 'die' naturally in the shops. They have been stripped of nutrients *so that* bacteria won't attack them. Far from being refined, they have been *destroyed*. A good general principle is to choose the most natural products possible.

- Wheat compromises our immune system, makes our body acidic, has a high Glycaemic Load and contributes little in terms of micronutrients.

- There is no nutritional requirement for sugar nor for hydrogenated and trans fats.

- Apart from foods that are obviously salty such as bacon and crisps, hidden salt can be found in many manufactured items, including bread, breakfast cereals, soup, canned food and most fast food.
- This chapter gives you a summary of some of the most recent information on nutrition. Reading at least one good book on nutrition will be helpful. The Notes for this chapter contain a number of suggestions, or perhaps you already have a good book you want to use. It's best to use books that focus on healthy eating rather than losing weight and looking good. If you don't know where to start, read the reader reviews for these books on the amazon.co.uk website to see which seem right for you.

NOTES

1   This is a good summary: 'A growing body of theoretical and experimental work suggests that diets designed to lower the insulin response to ingested carbohydrates may improve access to stored metabolic fuels, decrease hunger, and promote weight loss. Such a diet would contain abundant quantities of vegetables, fruits and legumes, moderate amounts of protein and healthful fats, and decreased intake of refined grain products, potato and concentrated sugars. Indeed, this diet bears a close resemblance to that consumed by human ancestors over the last several hundred thousand years.' *Journal of Nutrition* (2000) 130: 280S-283S, American Society for Nutritional Sciences; reprinted with permission.

2   There can be a significant difference between our chronological age and our biological age because the number of years since we were born doesn't necessarily relate to the condition of our body. For example, one very famous overeater, Elvis Presley, was said to have had the arteries of a man twice his age. In his 40s when he died, he had overeaten so much that his body reflected *a biological age of 80.*

3   In one study, 100 people were divided into two groups and compared for body composition using scanning technology. During the eight-week test, the experimental group consumed a whole-food nutritional supplement (*Juice Plus+®*) which meant they substantially increased their intake of fruits and vegetables, while the control group consumed a placebo. Both groups lost scale weight of about 1lb per week, but the experimental group had a far greater reduction in body fat and *gained* lean mass, thus achieving a threefold improvement in overall body composition. Moderate levels of exercise were the same in both groups. The study was published in the *Journal of the American Nutraceutical Association (1) 1998.*

4   It is now suggested that women with waists of more than 85 cm (34 inches) or more and men with waists of more than 99 cm (39 inches) or

more are at a higher risk of diabetes and heart disease. The larger your waist measurement, the higher your risk. As for your bodyfat percentage, it's best for men to stay between 12 to 18 per cent and for women to stay between 15 and 25 per cent, but not everyone has access to a way of measuring this.

5   A study of men and women aged between 87 and 96 resulted in tripled strength of leg muscles over a period of eight weeks, with associated improvements in their ability to walk. The study is mentioned in *Biomarkers: The 10 Keys to Prolonging Vitality* (Simon & Schuster, 1992).

6   'Revised International Table of Glycemic Index and Glycemic Load', *American Journal of Clinical Nutrition*, July 2002.

7   So many books have been written about the Glycaemic Index/Load, recommending one is very much a case of personal preference. *The South Beach Diet* by Dr Arthur Agatston (Headline, 2003) could be the easiest to understand and follow.

8   If much of this information on nutrition is new to you and you want to buy just one book to learn more, try *The pH Diet* by Bharti Vyas and Suzanne Le Quesne (Thorsons, 2004). It's specifically about balancing the pH of our bodies but it's an excellent all-round book on nutrition as well.

9   If I could read just one book on nutrition from now on, it would be *The Paleo Solution* by Robb Wolf (Victory Belt, 2010). The author is a former research biochemist and considered one of the world's leading experts in Paleolithic nutrition. His website at www.robbwolf.com has a vast amount of information too.

10 A BBC Panorama documentary (October, 2004) showed how a World Health Organization report which recommended sugar as part of a healthy diet had been secretly financed and strongly influenced by the sugar industry. Speaking on the programme, Dr Tim Lobstein, Director of the United Nations Food Commission, explained how the sugar industry works hard to undermine the credibility of sound science that

demonstrates the health risks of sugar. The massive amount of money at stake means that the Department of Health is continually lobbied and so backs off from making powerful statements about the danger to our health. Sounds like tobacco industry tactics to me!

11 It's often said that people eat commercially prepared food because it's less expensive, but in terms of nutritional value for money, you are much better off with food closer to its natural state. As a general principle, the more stages of processing a product has gone through – chopping, cooking, designing, packaging and marketing, all of which costs money – the less nutritional value you'll get. Notice that those cultures in our world today which have the most overweight populations are also the most affluent. Eating quantities of cheap, processed foods to 'fill yourself up' is doing nothing more than satisfying your addictive desire. Feeding most addictions is an expensive business, and food addiction can be one of the most costly to maintain.

CHAPTER 8

The Trouble with Hunger

When you're in a hole, the first thing to do is to stop digging.
ANON

When it comes to making changes in how much you eat, the most common advice is to eat only when you are genuinely hungry and to stop when you're full. At first glance this might seem good sense, but for many reasons – and for most overeaters – it is extremely unhelpful.

First of all, though, if it ain't broke, don't fix it! If it works for you to wait for natural hunger before you eat, that's great. And if you are someone who can tell when you've reached the right amount of fullness, by all means use that as your guide.

A great many people assume this is what they are supposed to be doing. However, because they continually fall short of this goal, they end up with a huge sense of hopelessness around the whole issue. The truth is that genuine body signals of hunger and fullness are often subtle and hard to read. As an obese client once said to me, 'I don't think I'd recognise natural hunger if it jumped up and bit me on the nose.'

These body signals can also be extremely confusing.

Many people seem to feel hungry *after* eating a meal. In fact, it's quite possible to conjure up some feelings of hunger almost any time at all. On the other hand, it's possible to go without eating for very long periods and still not feel any physical sensations of hunger. I have experienced this myself; I do not feel hungry, even though this makes no sense at all, considering when and how much I last ate. If you are waiting for hunger to appear, you could end up undereating, perhaps feeling faint and dizzy because you need food.

It's even more difficult to be sure you're 'full' – whatever that's supposed to mean! Most people don't feel the 'fullness' of what they ate until quite a few minutes after finishing a meal – *no matter what kind of food was consumed*. It's often said that it takes 20 minutes for that feeling of fullness to develop and if you tend to overeat, this is much too late. I bet you know as well as I do how much overeating can be done in 20 minutes! (1)

The truth is that sensations of hunger and fullness are not at all reliable. There'll be times when you'll feel hungry when you're really not and times when you won't feel hungry when you really are. This chapter will help you to sort it all out.

False Hunger

Many people start to feel false hunger when they try to reduce the amount they eat. Their overeating was masking the problem, and eating more appropriate amounts of food brings their false hunger to their attention. There are three different causes:

Stomach Acidity

This is often misinterpreted as natural hunger. However, natural hunger is never painful or unpleasant in any way. Stomach acidity feels painful, especially when your stomach is empty, so very understandably it makes it difficult to keep yourself from eating. Even the

> *The truth is that sensations of hunger and fullness are not at all reliable.*

possibility of feeling hungry later on can drive you to overeat rather than risk feeling the pain of an empty acid stomach.

I have struggled with stomach acidity in the past so I know what I'm talking about. I overate a lot in an attempt to get rid of the pain, but mostly I overate so that I wouldn't get hungry later on. Hunger hurt and sometimes it hurt a lot, especially in the middle of the night. That's what happens when you have an acid stomach.

Alcohol and coffee are common causes of stomach acidity and sometimes I notice that I seem to feel hungry soon after drinking a cup of coffee. I know I wouldn't have felt that hunger if I hadn't had the coffee. This is not hunger; it's a sign that my stomach has become a bit too acidic, and it's the acidity that's making me feel as if I'm hungry.

There are many kinds of antacid medication, but it's not a good idea to rely on them except in extreme cases when the acidity has become very distressing and, perhaps, an ulcer has already formed. It's much better to learn what's causing the problem in the first place. Eating alkaline-forming food has proved to be the most effective solution for me, together with regular exercise and very occasionally (during times of stress) a session of acupuncture. I still drink alcohol and coffee, but a great deal less than I used to. I find that moderate amounts aren't a problem as long as I take care to eat plenty of alkaline-forming foods.

As far as healthy eating goes, nutritionists advise us to balance 20 per cent acid-forming foods – meat, poultry, fish, eggs, grains and cheese – with 80 per cent alkaline-forming foods – most vegetables. As we saw in the previous chapter, over-acidity can lead to serious problems such as osteoporosis and arthritis (see page 140), so it's important to deal with this, quite apart from eliminating it as a cause of false hunger. The rewards I get from keeping my body more alkaline are lots of energy and being able to eat considerably less. (2)

Blood Glucose Levels

Our blood glucose levels rise and fall much too rapidly when we eat high-GL foods such as sugar, potatoes and processed grains (see page 137). Whenever our blood glucose levels fall too fast, we can start to feel hungry again. This kind of false hunger is called reactive hypoglycaemia – and it's very common.

A great deal has been written about this cause of false hunger and it is often claimed to be the sole cause of addictive overeating. Cut down or eliminate the high-GL carbs, they say, and you will eliminate your cravings for them. You now know that this is not the whole story, but the truth is that you will eliminate this source of false hunger – and that's not a bad result.

The basic principle is this: the more you eat the low-GL carbs (together with good fats and proteins) and the less you eat the high-GL carbs, the less false hunger you will feel. The low-GL foods are preferable, providing the body with a steady stream of energy and sustained mental alertness. If you are particularly susceptible to the rise and fall of blood glucose, it may be good to snack on low-GL food between meals as this will help to prevent the hypoglycaemic reaction. (3)

Addictive Hunger

This is the physical aspect of the addictive desire to eat. As we saw in Chapter 6, this addictive desire comes from your memory; it's the conditioned response to cues you have associated with food in the past. This response can be no more than a thought – but it can also be a strong sensation of false, addictive hunger or appetite.

A great deal of research over many years has shown that the conditioned response can cause the secretion of saliva in the mouth and digestive juices in the stomach, a drop in blood glucose levels and the release of dopamine in the brain – *all just at the thought of eating*. These physical effects could be fairly subtle but certainly noticeable. The conditioned response makes the body prepare for food intake, which is why it feels so much like real hunger, a genuine need for food. (4)

Addictive hunger will have an influence over when you are likely to *start* eating, but it also influences when you *stop* eating. It's very common for addictive hunger to surface during and at the end of a meal. The process of eating awakens your addictive appetite so that you end a meal wanting more – perhaps with even more of an appetite than you had when you started. This addictive, excessive appetite is often satisfied with another helping or two, another course, and/or by continuing to snack after your meal is finished.

It's also satisfied *in anticipation* by how much you serve yourself to begin with. In other words, you buy, cook and serve larger portions because you know that only this amount will satisfy you. When considering serving sizes, keep in mind that your stomach is supposed to be the size of your fist. Take into account that fruits and vegetables contain a high percentage of water, but know that some amount of your meal may be doing nothing but feeding and reinforcing your addictive hunger.

> **It's very common for addictive hunger to surface during and at the end of a meal.**

The meal often ends, not with an appropriate degree of fullness, but with some level of discomfort; feeling bloated, 'stuffed' and perhaps a bit disgusted with having eaten so much yet again. This is an 'aversive state' which turns off the addictive appetite. It can be quite subtle or extreme, but it's the same kind of aversive state some smokers get when they smoke too much at a party one night and don't feel much like smoking the following morning. This is a version of the 'crash' phase we looked at in Chapter 6, and many over-eaters go through this every day at every meal. The reason overeaters continue to go through this is because if that aversive state isn't reached, the addictive appetite isn't switched off and so *an unsatisfied addictive hunger remains*.

This is partly what's difficult about following the advice to 'stop when you're full' because it's all too easy to confuse 'feeling full' with 'feeling satisfied'. When you feel satisfied at the end of a meal, what's been satisfied is not just your natural hunger; it's also your addictive hunger.

Natural hunger is satisfied after the first few bites. I'm not suggesting that you only eat a few bites, just that your natural hunger will have been satisfied by then. If you only eat a couple of bites then your natural hunger will return very shortly. The feeling of not being satisfied at the end of a meal is your addictive hunger that wants to go on and on. You now know that you don't have to feed that hunger. You have a choice, and by choosing to leave it unsatisfied, you begin to lay it to rest.

In order to achieve your goal of eating less at meals, you will need to be willing to feel unsatisfied – *and not 'full'* – at the end of your meal. When you make a Plan before you start eating, you decide on a stopping point where you have the opportunity to confront your addictive hunger (see page 106). The last thing you want is a feeling of fullness and satisfaction. That's what got you into this problem in the first place!

Deprivation and Addictive Hunger

It's worth remembering here that an attitude of deprivation has the effect of exaggerating the addictive appetite. We saw in Chapter 5 that food actually tastes better when it seems less available (see page 83). And we looked at the 'Last Supper' effect, where overeating at meals occurs because of an underlying sense of deprivation (see page 89).

Research has demonstrated that animals will overeat when they have been trained to expect a particularly long wait before the next meal is delivered. You might think that they would be just as likely to overeat if it had been a long time since their last meal, but this is not the case! The most reliable way to get animals to overeat is to get them to anticipate a lengthy period of time with no food after the current meal. (5)

This sounds very much like being on a diet, but that dreadful state of deprivation can be created whether you're on a diet as such or not. It's simply the *thought* that you aren't going to be eating anything again for quite a while that drives overeating. The solution is not non-stop snacking; it's thinking in terms of free choice. Just keep your options open, remembering that you can always have something later on – and maybe you will!

Keeping your options open is the key. Your difficulty could be that if you always do have something later on (especially if it's a fairly considerable something) then you'll conclude that declaring 'no more food for me today' is the only way to get yourself to eat less. As you learn how to manage your addictive desire more effectively, however, you begin to trust yourself that having the *option* of eating later on isn't so dangerous after all. And by acknowledging that freedom, your addictive hunger – that grim determination to keep overeating while you still can – subsides.

Hunger, Hunger and Hunger

It's worth knowing that you can experience more than one – or all – of these hungers at the same time. You could have a natural hunger, an addictive hunger, stomach acidity and reactive hypoglycaemia all happening at once!

So what to do? First of all, it's very difficult and even unwise to keep yourself from eating if you have false hunger from stomach acidity and/or reactive hypoglycaemia. When you do eat, *eat in a way that rectifies the problem rather than exacerbates it*. By far the best response is to eat foods that keep your blood glucose balanced and your body more alkaline. Then you simply eliminate these causes of false hunger, leaving you with just your addictive and natural hunger. Both of these are going to be much easier to deal with when you aren't experiencing the other false hungers as well.

As for addictive hunger, use Times and Plans to help you identify it in the first place. Then, by thinking through The Outline and choosing to accept the feeling of unsatisfied desire, you gradually diminish it. If you choose your Times as you go, you can always get your meals and snacks to fit your schedule (see Chapter 6).

This is very important because waiting for natural hunger before you eat can be extremely inconvenient. If you are eating with others it's ridiculous to delay your meal until you are sure your hunger has appeared. And it isn't practical to skip a meal at lunchtime because you're not hungry, only to find you are hungry an hour or two later during a shift at work, in a meeting or when you need to pick the kids up from school.

It makes sense to aim for natural hunger as a sign to eat, but by setting Times you have a guideline that's more tangible and therefore less easily misinterpreted. Even more important, it's completely flexible to suit your schedule.

At least to begin with, it would be best to choose your food from an intellectual understanding based on your best assessment of the advice given. If, after some time, you are no longer overeating, you are eating only natural food, and you are moving your body around as nature intended – *then* you might expect natural and reliable body signals that let you know when to start and stop eating. Think of 'eating when hungry and stopping when full' as goals to aim towards, rather than tools to help you gain control of overeating.

Even so, you are still likely to experience some amount of addictive hunger and will all too easily come up with a host of wonderful reasons as to why you should satisfy it. This is the subject of the next two chapters.

IN OTHER WORDS: KATH

I heard someone say on the radio recently that the reason people eat too much is because they are bored. I can absolutely say that for me at least this is completely wrong because I am the mother of three children, all under six, so boredom doesn't happen in my life at all.

My overeating was all done at two times of the day, pretty much every day. Around 4 o'clock in the afternoon was a big one for me, and in the evening when the kids had got to sleep. I didn't have any difficulty at any other time, but at those times it was mad. I just ate and ate, always comfort food, anything I could find that was bread or sugary, and I would just think, 'I deserve it, this is something for me.' I would have spent the day driving the children to and from places, looking out for them, feeding them, whatever, and then a moment or two would appear in my day and it would be TIME FOR ME!

When I talked it through with Gillian two things stood out most for me. The main thing was becoming aware of how much I thought in terms of prohibition. I just hadn't realised how much I monitored my life with 'I've got to' and 'I mustn't' and very much feeling that I'm not allowed to snack, binge, overeat . . . to be naughty! When I was growing up, my mother controlled my every move, and I ➤

can feel her even now in my head telling me what I must and must not do. Understanding this has been such a big breakthrough for me. Now when I hear mother's voice, I usually just shout back at her (in my head, not out loud).

The other thing that's helped me a lot is noticing which kinds of food satisfy me for longer and which are likely to have me reaching for more food very soon. For example, I've switched to a rye bread and more veggies at lunchtime, and now my energy lasts through the afternoon. This means I'm not so fraught at that 4 o'clock time, and it's making more sense to eat something wholesome to keep me going until dinner. It has an effect on my energy and also my mood and how patient I am with the kids. So I've made these changes FOR ME, because I'm seeing real benefits that I want for myself.

Taking Control

- Just because you're naturally hungry, this doesn't mean you're not about to eat in an addictive way. To take extreme examples, there are plenty of people who regularly eat a packet of biscuits, or crisps or cake for dinner. They are feeding their natural hunger but what they're doing is entirely addictive.

- If you fear feeling natural hunger, just make sure you have immediate access to food. It would be a good idea to keep real, natural food around, though, and not addictive snacks. This doesn't necessarily mean that you should go ahead and eat at the first sign of hunger; just knowing that you could *will make all the difference.*

- Whenever you microwave any food you make it more acidic. Microwaving or boiling also destroys live enzymes (which detoxify the body), folic acid and almost all the antioxidants in vegetables and fruit.

- Exercise makes your body more alkaline, as does deep breathing and any form of stress reduction, such as meditation or yoga.

- Foods should not be regarded either as healthy or unhealthy on their Glycaemic Load alone (see page 137). It's just one factor of many, and certainly fat content should also be taken into consideration. The problem for many of us is that we have eaten too many high-GL carbs too often.

NOTES

1   Many published studies confirm the unreliability of perceivable sensations of hunger. One paper on research at the University of London concludes '. . . there is no strong and characteristic pattern of hunger symptoms.' *British Journal of Clinical Psychology* 1987; 26 153–4.

As for the reliability of 'fullness', in my book, *Willpower!* (Vermilion, 2003), I describe a study by Paul Rozin of the University of Pennsylvania involving two men with severe short-term memory loss. The men were given lunch and offered another soon after. Because they had no memory of having already eaten, they consumed THREE substantial, three-course meals before refusing a fourth!

And according to Dr Andrew Prentice, as Head of Obesity Research at the MRC Dunn Clinical Nutrition Centre, 'Physiological studies show that human metabolism is very poorly adapted to recognise excess fat consumption.' *British Medical Bulletin* 1997; 53, 229–237, by permission of Oxford University Press.

2   See *The pH Diet* by Bharti Vyas and Suzanne Le Quesne (Thorsons, 2004) for clear explanations on the link between over-acidity and osteoporosis, osteoarthritis, rheumatoid arthritis and gout. Back pain, frozen shoulder and tennis elbow can also be associated.

3   See *The South Beach Diet* by Dr Arthur Agatston (Headline, 2003).

4   'The conditioning process generates a conditioned response to the conditioned stimulus which is biologically similar to the state we think of as "real" hunger . . . salivation, hyperinsulinaemia, increased release of gastric peptides, increased gut mobility, and so on.' Reprinted from *Addictive Behaviors* 15, Wardle, J, 387–393(1990) with permission from Elsevier.

5   '... the animal appears to be eating in order to last until food will be available again.' Reprinted from *Addictive Behaviors* (see above).

CHAPTER 9

Your Reasons Why

I always keep a stimulant handy in case I see a snake — which I also keep handy.
W.C. FIELDS

This is a good chapter to use for troubleshooting. You may just want to dip in and out of it whenever you find you are feeding your addictive desire to eat a bit too often. What you want to look for are the ways in which you are justifying your overeating. One way to do this is to delay satisfying your addictive desire until you have spotted the justification. There always is one.

The justification may flash through your mind faster than lightning: 'I'm going to go ahead and eat this because . . .' It may be because you'll enjoy it or because it will comfort you when you feel miserable. Maybe you want to join in with others or it's because you feel bored. Or perhaps you think 'I'd better finish it off before it goes bad'. The desire always wants to be satisfied, *and our addiction will automatically select the most plausible, sensible and reasonable justification available at the time.*

The justifications often lurk at the back of our minds, not completely recognised. They encourage our overeating, but when they are not clearly identified they cannot be brought out into the open for examination. On examination, your justifications could be sound ones you wish to continue to use. Some might contain kernels of truth but be of questionable use at times. Some may serve no purpose at all other than to insist that you eat.

Call them reasons, justifications, explanations or excuses. You justify *how much* you are about to eat, *how often* you eat and the *quality* of what you eat. You don't necessarily need to judge these reasons as 'right' or 'wrong'. Some could be appropriate in some circumstances but not in others.

If you eat quite a bit more food than your body needs, you are too attached to too many of these reasons too often. So, instead of creating the results you want, *you live with the reasons why you couldn't manage to succeed.*

Determine which of these justifications serve you and which block your way. Only when you are aware of your reasons for eating can you freely choose which reasons you want to use. Then, you could aim to use them within the structure of Times and Plans (see page 105).

It's essential to have some reason to justify eating! Someone with anorexia may not accept any at all, even the risk of dying from malnutrition. But you don't *have to* eat in response to any of your reasons. It's always your choice as to whether or not you satisfy any desire to eat, addictive or not.

There's any number of justifications, and some may be unique to you. It's very possible that you have used some justifications for much of your life and have little or no personal experience of how invalid they really are. Here are some of the most typical, with suggestions about how to let go of them.

I'm Eating This Because . . .

Habit and Tradition

'*I always eat cornflakes for breakfast*', '*I always eat popcorn at the cinema*', '*It's the way I was brought up*', '*We always eat pizza on Thursdays*', '*I always finish a meal with something sweet*', '*I always eat something as soon as I get home*'. It is possible to eat according to your traditions within the structure of Times and Plans. It's also possible to recognise and accept the addictive desire which is associated with a particular circumstance, routine or time of day. Habit plays a significant role in any addiction. It's not the complete explanation for addiction, but it's a part of the picture. People who stop smoking experience their addictive desire in exactly the same way. For example, they feel their desire to smoke as they leave their office, if it was their habit to smoke then.

To take control of your addictive eating, you don't need to change the routines with which it is associated. That will be impossible in most cases anyway. For example, you might buy a chocolate bar whenever you buy a newspaper at the corner shop. Unless you move to the North Pole you won't be able to avoid corner shops. Just expect to feel your addictive desire in those circumstances, especially at first. It will help to use The Outline (see page 126).

Be careful of justifying eating food because it is traditional or ethnic. A kind of food associated with a religious or racial group could still have the nutrition processed out of it and bad fats added.

And notice that you could be just as likely to justify feeding your addictive desire by something outside of your everyday routine, such as a holiday. The conditioned response can be associated with things that don't happen very often, such as the seasons. You might have trained yourself to eat more when the days get shorter, for example.

Stress

'I always overeat when I'm stressed', *'I've had such a hard day at work'*, *'I need to relax'*. Far from alleviating the problem, addictive eating actually makes you more stressed. High-GL carbs in particular cause more stress hormones to be released. Stress causes the body to become more acidic, so acid-forming foods such as sugar and wheat aggravate that as well. Both stress and addictive eating impair your immune system. And when you are stressed your digestive system is less efficient, so during stressful times it's wiser to eat lighter and more natural food.

Exercise, relaxation techniques such as yoga, meditation and autogenic training, and cutting down on stimulants such as caffeine and sugar are far more effective responses to stress.

This is where you can really see addiction at work, because the chances are you will not want to regard these as viable alternatives. Your addictive thinking latches on to the best reason to snack on biscuits and coffee, not the best reason for a long walk! The difference between your level of interest in genuine solutions versus overeating could be seen as a measure of your addiction to food.

You can only break down the conditioned response in the circumstances where it occurs, so it's only when you're stressed that you can make real changes. Don't avoid stress (as if you could!), and remember it's always your choice to feed and reinforce your addiction or manage your addictive desire. Then you could discover new strategies that really help you to relax. (1)

Physical Wellbeing

'I don't feel too well', 'I have a headache', 'I'm cold'. Any physical ailment, upset, ache or pain can be a cue for an addictive desire, simply because in the past you have conditioned yourself to eat in response to such things. This does not necessarily mean that eating would be an appropriate response. All it may mean is you are experiencing your addictive desire again.

> **Your addictive thinking latches on to the best reason to snack on biscuits and coffee, not the best reason for a long walk!**

'I'm constipated'. The best cure is not eating more but exercise and plenty of water – and avoiding the fibre-free processed foods that create the problem in the first place. If you tend to suffer from constipation, notice which foods you have been eating and learn by trial and error. Also, there are very good natural remedies, such as aloe vera, acidophilus supplements and linseeds, available from health food shops.

'I'm premenstrual'. When you understand that addictive desire is a memory, you can see that it can be associated with all kinds of physical states. The physical shifts that occur at times during the menstrual cycle could be obvious or subtle, even imperceptible, but can often trigger an addictive desire associated with this time of the month. All it takes is having eaten in an addictive way at this time in the past. Far from alleviating the problems of PMS, addictive eating makes it much worse. Several books have been written on this subject. (2)

'I'm tired and need a pick-me-up'. This could be a very important reason to eat something – or it could be one of your favourite excuses for addictive eating. The way to tell the difference is to see whether you really do get more energy after you've eaten something, and this can be learned only by trial and error. If you feel dizzy or tired, and then perk up when you eat, this indicates that you have been undereating. Either it's been way too long since you ate something, or what you last ate was of poor nutritional quality. If you sincerely suspect you have undereaten, *eat something immediately*. This is a valid reason to eat before your Time.

This assumes that you aren't perking yourself up with artificial stimulants such as sugar, wheat, chocolate or caffeine. All high-GL carbs give us a burst of energy because they stimulate the release of adrenaline, which is partly why they are so addictive. The energy they provide is brief, though, and afterwards we are worse off – more tired, stressed and undernourished.

Natural Hunger

'I'm starving', *'I'm really hungry'*, *'I might get hungry later on'*. A feeling of emptiness in your stomach, natural hunger is one of the best reasons to eat, although it's not a reliable signal for everyone. Sometimes I eat when I'm naturally hungry and sometimes I don't. What's important is I don't fear it. If you fear natural hunger, you'll continue to overeat.

Your body isn't harmed by feeling hungry sometimes. It's only your addictive thinking that objects, especially that state of deprivation you create when you deny choice. Some amount of natural hunger is actually beneficial to you because it means your body isn't loaded down with food to digest. Digestion is one of the most demanding tasks your body performs, so natural hunger means your body is relaxing instead of being overworked. Your body feels lighter and has more energy and vitality, and your mind is more alert. And because you're not overeating, your self-esteem is higher, too.

Natural hunger should be a pleasant and even enjoyable sensation which just comes and goes. There should be nothing uncomfortable about it. It may be hard to believe at first, but in time, as you work through your addictive thinking, you can actually enjoy feeling some natural hunger every day.

Social

'Everybody is eating this and I want to join in', *'Eating is a way to be social'*, *'It would be rude not to accept it'*, *'I'll eat a lot to show it's appreciated'*. Notice how often you let other people dictate the quality, quantity and frequency of your eating. At times it may be appropriate – but not always. It's essential for you to be able to say, at least sometimes, 'No thanks' or 'Can I save it for later?' And it's important for you to be able to do that and feel okay about it. You can assert yourself in a polite and sensitive way, and other people may not be as offended as your addiction wants you to imagine!

Be aware, though, that others may, perhaps unconsciously, try to sabotage you. It's likely that the people around you eat addictively, and your addictive eating helps them justify theirs. They may fear change in you, and not fully understand what's going on.

'I only have a good time if I'm overeating'. If you forget you are making choices and why you are making them, you can

feel deprived (miserable, envious and martyred) if you are eating less than usual or less than everyone else. If you deal effectively with your addictive thinking you'll be able to enjoy eating less – and still enjoy the company and the good food.

'I must eat it now while it's still available'. This is really saying 'I'll eat it now while I still can, because I won't be able to later.' Instead, give yourself permission to eat it now and permission to eat it at any time in the future. If someone offers me something gorgeous, and I see eating it as addictive, it will be much easier for me to say 'no' if I allow myself the possibility of eating some later. If I still want it, I can include it or something like it in my next Plan.

Pleasure and satisfaction

'It looks so good I have to have some', *'I enjoy my food'*, *'Food is my hobby, my career and/or the love of my life'*, *'I won't feel satisfied unless I have more'*. Remember that pleasure is an integral part of addiction. The smoker, drug addict and alcoholic all pursue immediate pleasure, and in doing so value it more highly than their health and self-esteem. This is what you do too, when you eat addictively.

As an overeater, you confuse the appropriate pleasure and satisfaction everybody gets from eating with the satisfaction of your addictive desire. The tools of Times and Plans will help you learn how to distinguish between your natural and addictive appetites. When you use The Outline to make fewer and fewer choices to feed the addictive desire, you can derive enormous pleasure from eating less – in a guilt-free, non-addictive way. This is consistent with good health and strong self-esteem.

Deprivation

'I don't want to miss out', 'I deserve it', 'It's my reward', 'I don't want to deprive myself', 'I'm no good at self-denial'. If this is the theme of your justifications, it indicates that you have not yet fully owned a real sense of choice about eating. This is very common. It's something you can change and when you do it makes a big difference. Whenever you notice yourself using this type of justification, the key is to remind yourself that you've got choices and what the consequences of different choices are.

> **The smoker, drug addict and alcoholic all pursue immediate pleasure, and in doing so value it more highly than their health and self-esteem.**

These justifications focus on the food and your desire for that food, not the whole picture. The whole picture would include the consequences to your health, energy and self-esteem. Only when you feel free to choose whatever you want, can you just as easily believe: 'I don't want to miss out on good health', 'I deserve more energy' and 'My reward is my sense of achievement and peace of mind'. The only difference in making those choices is that your addictive desire doesn't get satisfied.

As for missing out, I've found it helpful to accept that there will always be an extraordinary amount of fabulous food in the world that I will never get to eat. When I accept that I cannot possibly eat *all* of it, I can start to let go of more and more of it.

'I can't be bothered', 'I'll start again tomorrow'. Whenever you come up against this justification for overeating, remind yourself that you don't *have to* do anything. Let that sink in by picturing your life without making any changes at all.

Then, if you have any motivation to change, it will become apparent and you'll want to be bothered to make the effort that's required.

Nutrition

'I haven't had enough protein/vitamin C/iron today', *'I don't know much about nutrition, so I'd better eat a lot to make sure I get enough of what I need'*. When you make your health your priority, you have the best motivation there is to eat lower-quantity and higher-quality food. A substantial amount of research supports this. The way to improve your immune system, slow down the aging process and live a longer and healthier life is to choose a wide variety of foods of the highest possible nutritional value – and not to eat too much. (3)

'I'm pregnant so I'm eating for two'. It's possible that pregnancy will throw your eating off balance for all sorts of reasons. Take your doctor's advice as to how rapid your weight gain should be. If you are gaining too much weight too quickly, perhaps you have discovered another justification for addictive overeating.

Denial

'It's just a little tiny bit, just this once', *'I eat less than my skinny friends'*, *'I have a slow metabolism'*, *'I put on weight if I just look at a piece of chocolate'*. One of the most compelling reasons to overeat is to convince yourself that you are not overeating at all. Denial is common to all addictions at some point. Smokers say 'I'd quit if it ever affected my health.' Alcoholics say 'I never drink alone, so I don't have a problem.' It's one of the most powerful ways for an addiction to justify itself.

There's quite a bit of research on obesity that shows how

common it is to underestimate amounts consumed. Overweight subjects are asked to write down everything they eat in a day, but researchers discover the discrepancy when they compare these records with an analysis of urine samples which shows how many calories have in fact been consumed. It's entirely possible the subjects don't deliberately intend to mislead. They are simply in the habit of fooling themselves into believing they eat less and aren't even aware they are overeating. According to a great deal of research into this issue, slim and overweight volunteers, fed the same restricted diet, all lose weight in an entirely predictable way. When energy intake is below energy requirements then – and only then – people lose weight. (4)

'*I was born fat, it's just the way I am*'. Some people believe they just happen to be overweight, no matter what they do. This means they can avoid facing the reality of their overeating, making them less likely to consider how much they eat every day, and to recognise the amount of sugar, wheat, fat and salt they consume as the real cause of their problem.

'*I have a very healthy diet*'. We can also delude ourselves into believing we eat the highest-quality, healthiest diet, when in fact we don't. Very often a few token adjustments are made, and we use this to convince ourselves we eat wisely. Then this is used to justify satisfying any addictive desire: 'I normally eat such healthy food, a few biscuits won't make a difference.' Perhaps it won't, but do notice how frequently you use this justification to choose poor-quality food. There have been times when I've used it every day!

Waste

'It's wrong to throw away food when there are so many hungry people in the world', 'Today is its "best by" date, so I'd better finish it off now', 'I'll eat the leftovers, so they won't be wasted'. But surely one of the most tragic examples of wasted food is overeating! There are people starving in this world, but eating addictively is hardly a solution. Throwing food away can be a very constructive thing for you to do because it sends such a powerful message to your addiction: this is better off in the bin than in my stomach! It's only your addictive thinking that will tell you otherwise.

Convenience

'I don't have time to cook so I'll get my meal at the super-market/the chip shop/the takeaway', 'I'm at the chip shop, so there's only fried foods to choose from'. Your choices about what you are going to eat are made at least in part at the shop when you decide what to buy, and even in choosing which shop to go to. The same applies in choosing a restaurant because you know what you're likely to eat at each particular place, be it Chinese food, McDonalds or the pizza place with the salad bar.

Take note if you're justifying eating poor-quality food by telling yourself you have limited options at the burger bar or that you don't have time to do any better. It's likely you are playing the 'Why Don't You, Yes But' game. Good-quality food is available if you really want to find it.

Doing badly

'I already blew it so I might as well keep eating'. This usually comes from years of dieting which creates the cycle of compliance and rebellion described in Chapter 5. You may find it difficult to regain control once you've given it up, but stopping at any point is always an improvement. Simply set a Time, preferably between one and four hours ahead (see page 106). If becoming rebellious about eating is common for you, study Chapter 5, working on the exercises at the end, especially the last two.

'I'm too busy to deal with this', 'I've got so much to cope with in my life, I can't possibly think about dealing with my addiction as well'. Tell yourself the truth: your overeating takes up time, thought and energy too. Making choices to accept your feeling of desire doesn't take a great deal of time, and some of your rewards will be greater alertness, less stress and feeling more on top of things in general due to stronger self-esteem and improved health.

Doing Well

'I've lost some weight so it's okay to eat a bit more'. This justification is the main cause of yo-yo dieting. If losing weight is your priority (perhaps the only reason you don't satisfy your addictive desire) then *your motivation disappears along with the weight.* So the more attached you are to weight loss, the more likely you are to put the weight back on! When you care a bit less about your body size and shape, and more about the benefits you gain from higher self-esteem – especially from caring about your health as a preventative measure – staying in control of your eating will continue to motivate you.

'I've burned off about 400 calories at the gym so I can eat a Mars bar and still be ahead'. This means that weight loss is

still your main motivation. Counting calories has nothing to do with taking control of addictive eating. Not only that, but counting calories doesn't always lead to weight loss, because it depends on what kind of food the calories come from.

'I've been so good I deserve it'. What you may really be saying is 'I'm doing so well, I'd better screw it up'. If you have low self-esteem, success at anything will tend to feel odd, and you may get drawn into sabotaging yourself just so you feel 'your normal self' again. This is why it's so important to work on self-esteem along with taking control of your eating. *It's crucial that you esteem yourself enough to be able to tolerate your success.*

'I might become anorexic'. Anorexia and bulimia are characterised by low self-esteem, a strong fear of weight gain, wildly out-of-control bingeing and starving, and an obsession with food and dieting. Some of you may identify with these, but not as a result of reading this book and using Times, Plans and The Outline (see pages 105–9, 126). Long-term overeaters could not develop anorexia or bulimia simply as a result of learning how to manage their addictive appetite.

When you apply the techniques in this book, the amounts you end up eating may seem alarmingly small, but only in comparison to what you used to eat. The truth is we don't need very much food in order to stay in good health, provided our food is of high nutritional quality. (5)

False Self-identity

'I am an overeater, therefore I overeat', *'I'm hopeless'*, *'I have no willpower'*. We all create false beliefs about ourselves – usually based on only one or two experiences at first – and

then act in accordance with those beliefs over and over again, thus 'proving' their validity. When it comes to eating, it will help you to separate such beliefs from the truth. Addictive behaviour is always supported by lies. Telling the truth is the way to take control.

For example, it may be true when you say 'I eat addictively at times', but when you make this mean something else like 'I have no willpower', that's not the truth. The truth here is more likely to be 'Right now I'm not using my willpower to take control of my addictive eating', and when you put it like that you can see there's the possibility of making a change.

Watch out especially for all those ways you describe yourself as inadequate. *Your biggest obstacle to taking control of your eating could be your lack of belief in your ability to do it.* This is usually rooted in convictions such as 'I'm too old, fat, lazy, weak, self-indulgent, busy and/or stupid'.

Underlying beliefs such as these don't disappear in an instant, but it really will help you to remember that nothing about life is ever static. Change may happen slowly, even imperceptibly, but things will change. The first time you refuse to use your negative beliefs as a justification for overeating you probably won't experience anything like a life-enhancing transformation, but if you continue to do that, in time that's exactly what you'll achieve!

Past Hurts

'I overeat because of my unhappy childhood/my parents' divorce/my divorce'. Painful experiences in the past, an unhappy or even less-than-perfect childhood often provide a constantly available justification for any addiction you choose. Many addicts blame their past, claiming it's the reason they are the way they are today.

Alcoholics Anonymous tackles this issue by directing attention not to the past injustice, which of course can never be changed, but to the alcoholic's continued resentment of the people involved. Begin to let go of your resentment, they advise, and you begin to heal yourself. Alcoholics who stay sober through AA don't need to approve of past hurts, just to forgive and – crucial in this process – to refuse to use whatever happened as a justification for drinking.

After all, it's not what happened in your life that creates the problem; it's the fact that you use what happened to justify overeating. You have your explanation about why you overeat and you tell it to yourself over and over again: 'This happened to me – and that's why I'm eating again.' What matters *now* is not the past but how you are justifying your overeating *now*.

Your justifications, of course, are all going to be attached to your addictive desire to eat; it's only when you have an addictive desire that you'll justify satisfying it. Your addictive desire could have been developed during a time of emotional trauma, such as a divorce, but the desire often remains long after the trauma is over. This is often a source of confusion. I've heard clients say that they know they have worked through and resolved past difficulties, and are left wondering why they continue to overeat.

'*Addictive overeating represses emotions*', '*Whenever I try to diet I get irritable and depressed*', '*I can't cope if I'm not overeating*'. When people start to take control of their overeating, they are often more in touch with their feelings, both joyful and painful. However, most people try to eat less with an attitude that creates symptoms of deprivation, so it's common to experience more extreme negative moods. As a result it can certainly seem that overeating is the only way to maintain a happy life and acceptable personality. These feelings, however, are not repressed emotions coming to the surface, but very understandable and appropriate reactions to the denial of choice.

If you identify with this, increase your sense of free choice and the bad moods will evaporate. Then you discover that there is no monster lurking beneath the surface of your consciousness. You simply feel more alive and more in touch with feelings of joy and enthusiasm as well as entirely appropriate feelings of sadness and anger.

Present Upsets

'I'm feeling sad and if I eat something I'll feel better', *'I eat whenever I feel bored/lonely/depressed'*, *'Eating helps me cope when I feel bad'*. Also common, of course, is to use current emotional states to justify addictive eating. The key here is to remember that the conditioned response of addictive desire is triggered by mood states (such as feeling angry) just as easily as circumstances (such as watching television). So, first of all expect to feel your addictive desire to eat in all the situations where you ate in the past, especially if you ate addictive food. Of course it can be challenging to manage your addictive desire to eat during a period of low mood, whatever it is and whatever the cause. But it's only when you start to make choices to accept the inevitable desire and not act on it that you can find out for yourself *what it's like to experience that mood without overeating*.

In many different ways, overeating doesn't really help

you cope with your life at all. If anything, it makes life more difficult for you. It makes life more difficult because consuming too much processed and refined food contributes to poor nutrition, and this is often an underlying cause of depression, stress and low energy. Research has shown that people who improve their nutritional intake usually feel stronger emotionally as a result. (6)

Addictive eating also makes life more difficult because of the tendency to identify emotions as a hunger and nothing else. This inevitably results in some degree of emotional dishonesty, such as when you pretend you're happy when really you're angry. In choosing to accept your addictive hunger you choose to sober up. You become more in touch with your true feelings and therefore more authentic. (7)

Most of all, addictive eating makes life more difficult because of the effect it has on your self-esteem. There's no doubt that the stronger your self-esteem, the better you will be able to cope with whatever it is life throws at you. Remember this as you make your choices at these tough times and you will be able to begin to break those conditioned associations. Then you'll just have emotions coming and going like anyone else, and won't be so drawn to food.

Whenever you feel upset and want to eat, you could spend some time simply allowing yourself to feel your feelings, asking yourself what you can learn from or do about this particular situation. It's that immediate, urgent, addictive desire that gets triggered by your feelings that's the most beneficial to accept.

Also, notice just how miserable you need to feel in order to use feeling bad as a justification. Is it simply the ups and downs of daily life? It's not that eating won't or shouldn't cheer you up sometimes; it's just that this easily becomes your excuse for any eating at all. It's one thing to feel comforted by a bowl of good soup when you're tired and hungry, but quite another to eat junk food all morning because you woke up a bit grumpy.

> *Through repetition, a path is worn in the brain to activate our addictive desire – and any relevant excuse will suffice.*

This doesn't mean your feelings are not important, but addictive eating is not the answer. It's likely that you aren't addicted to the real solutions, so they won't hold the same appeal. Counselling, a good recovery or personal development programme and/or physical activity need cost no more than the amount of time and money you are currently spending on food you don't need. For many people, these strategies will be an important part of taking control of overeating. (8)

Many people explain addictive eating entirely in terms of covering up negative emotional states. But our addictive thinking automatically selects the most plausible justification available, so a happy moment of celebration can become an equally compelling excuse to overeat. If our behaviour was guided by our wanting to avoid feelings and nothing else, then going for a run would do just as well! But most of us don't even think of doing some physical exercise when we feel upset. I'm not suggesting it as a solution necessarily; my point is that whenever you feel strong emotions, two things are going on: your feelings and your conditioned response to those feelings, which is your addictive desire.

Addiction isn't just about avoiding unpleasant and unwanted feelings. It's a strong association that has been reinforced, probably for years, with those feelings. Through repetition, a path is worn in the brain to activate our addictive desire – and any relevant excuse will suffice.

If Only

'If only I had a different job, if only I had a man/woman in my life, if only I lived in my own flat, if only my family were less demanding, if only I had a different man/woman in my life, if only my life was more interesting, if only I lived in a different country . . . then I'd be able to take control of my addictive eating'. Regrets or disappointments are often used to justify addictions. When you think about something you regret, you'll feel your addictive desire to eat, through association, if you ate addictively in response to those thoughts in the past.

If you want a reason to keep overeating, you'll *always* be able to find one. Alternatively, you could make some different decisions about one thing you have complete choice about: what and how much you eat. Then, as a direct result you will be able to view the other circumstances in your life in a new way.

Once you start to own your choices about overeating, you'll begin to recognise your choices about other things too. Although many of these things may depend at least partly on other people's actions – which you are not responsible for – you will be able to see more clearly what choices you have. And you will be motivated by higher self-esteem to take the actions that are required. But even if nothing else changes in your life, at least you will be in control of your overeating, and that's no small thing.

If your 'if only . . .' justification has anything to do with not having enough money, remember what happened to

Ernie Bailey! He won £11 million on the lottery and barely stopped eating, drinking and smoking until he died of a heart attack 20 months later, weighing 22 stone. (9)

Addictions tend to persist, despite the circumstances. You're likely to want to eat addictively when you're lonely *and* when you're surrounded by friends. When you're bored *and* when you're busy. When you're in your daily routines *and* when you're off on holiday. Taking control of addiction, despite the circumstances, is powerful and liberating – and could well be the only effective strategy you can take.

Comfort Eating

'Food is love', *'Food is a friend who comforts me'*, *'I eat and I feel better'*. The three previous sections could also be described as comfort eating, which is said to be the most common justification given for addictive overeating. It's going to be tough, if not impossible, to deal with this unless you approach it with a genuine sense of choice. Start by fully choosing to comfort yourself by overeating and know that you can continue to do that. You are allowed! Then – and only then – you can gain a perspective that includes the downside. (If there is no downside, by the way, there is no problem.) Choose the downside as well, and you'll get in touch with your motivation to make different choices.

Body Wisdom

'I crave some foods because I'm allergic to them'. An allergy is the body's immune response to something it thinks is a potential threat. The most common food allergies are thought to be to dairy products and wheat, and it could be

that you are allergic to these or other kinds of food. However, an explanation of allergy as a *cause* of addiction is insufficient as it doesn't explain why an allergy to cats, for example, produces an aversion, when an allergy to wheat is said to produce an attraction. The connection between allergy and addiction is that overeating addictive foods such as wheat creates an allergic, toxic reaction after a period of time, rather than the other way around.

Once you know which foods you are allergic to, you can certainly end up with a more problematic attraction to that food if you then think 'Now I can't eat that any more'. But that's because of the way you are thinking about it – denying choice and then rebelling against that – not because of the biochemistry involved.

'I have a sweet tooth'. No you don't. You have an addictive desire for a drug known as refined sugar. The only connection this has with your teeth is that eating sugar promotes tooth decay. This common justification provides a good insight into how insidious this addiction is, because so much in our culture makes it seem normal.

'My body knows I need chocolate, bread, peanuts, bananas, etc.' This is another popular justification for overeating. For example, a friend of mine says that every so often she feels compelled to eat quite a lot of French bread. She explains this to me by saying there must be some nutrient in this bread that her body requires, and so she feels 'a need' for it.

You too may use this reason to justify either the quality or the quantity of what you eat – but do you ever use 'body wisdom' as a reason *not* to eat something? After all, if your body is that wise, why doesn't it stop you overeating? It doesn't do this because what you call your body's signal of nutritional need is more likely to be your addictive desire to eat.

A client told me a similar story, with the same explanation, with rice cakes instead of the French bread. Both French bread and rice cakes are high-GL carbs. They cause insulin to be released into the bloodstream very rapidly, and so are more likely to be eaten addictively.

This is a very common theme I encounter with clients, who often talk about listening to their body as if they are deciphering messages about what they need to eat. Some books promote this idea too, suggesting, for example, that a desire for chocolate is your body's way of telling you that you need magnesium.

Now, if this system really worked, *no one would ever be deficient in any nutrients.* As soon as people were low in iron or calcium or whatever, they would immediately crave the food they needed – spinach or kale, for example – and correct the problem. Your body might know what it needs but that message can only be received via your mind, and your mind is influenced by addiction. This means you will experience relentless and automatic justifications for overeating.

Remember, too, that people around you are probably overeaters to some degree as well, so these things will also apply to them. Just because they believe, for example, that sugar is a valuable source of energy doesn't necessarily make it true. Human beings survived for many thousands of years before refined sugar was created. We don't need to fear the disease and famine which killed off our ancestors at an early age. We have our present-day epidemic of addiction to contend with.

One final point. There is an entirely different way you can

listen to your body, and this is to observe physical states and sensations *after* having eaten. Are you lethargic and bloated or full of energy and vitality? The changes in these states might be quite subtle, but by all means keep noticing them and the foods associated with them. Pay attention to your body's excess weight, symptoms of ill health, headaches and low energy. In this sense, your body is clearly trying to tell you something important.

Justifying Weight

'My excess fat protects me from the world', 'my weight keeps me from getting unwanted attention from the opposite sex'. Remember from Chapter 2 that weight is an effect, not a cause, of your problem. Imagine someone trying to justify smoking by claiming some advantage to spending each morning coughing! Smokers have developed an addictive desire for cigarettes, not for coughing. As an overeater, you have developed an addictive desire for food, not for weight. There are plenty of other ways to protect yourself and to avoid unwanted attention from the opposite sex, such as wearing baggy, unfashionable clothing.

'It's middle-age spread'. This could be true in part, but just a little part. Some experts say we can reasonably expect to gain about 5lb for each decade after 20 – assuming we weren't overweight at 20, in which case we could lose weight as we age. We need less food as we get older, so if we eat less – responding to our physical needs rather than our addiction – we will find that the all-too-common weight gain is not at all inevitable. (10)

Exercise, of course, also plays an important part. Many people gain weight as they age simply because they become less active. If we eat just enough to meet our nutritional needs but don't exercise, we will gain weight. A lack of physical activity is one of the most important factors in obesity and its associated health problems.

'*My parents were fat too, so it must be my genes*'. Of course we inherit many features from our family gene pool, but we still have our own choices about how we live. For example, we don't have to have the same political views as our parents or the same taste in clothes. Our genes might dictate what part of our body our weight goes on, but our genes do not preside over our eating choices and therefore do not have the final word about how much weight we will carry. (11)

Genes are often blamed for all addictive behaviours, but the same principle applies. *You may have been born with a genetic predisposition to become addicted, but you always have free choice as to whether or not you will continue to satisfy and reinforce your addiction.*

IN OTHER WORDS: MARGHERITA

Treating eating as an addiction was a difficult concept to grasp at first – after all, you have to eat a certain amount to live. But once you learn to recognise the addictive desire as separate from 'normal' eating, so many things fall into place. All those excuses and justifications you've used for years fall away, and the simple acceptance that I EAT TOO MUCH is wonderfully liberating.

I now look at things like ice cream and chocolates and think 'I can eat that if I want to'. But now I am thinking about what I eat and getting into the habit of choosing ➤

> the longer-term good of my body and self-esteem over
> the short-term moment of pleasure in the mouth – and it's
> a great feeling.
>
> The technique of Times and Plans is especially useful
> for the evening meal, I find, as it keeps me from nibbling
> before and after dinner, when I'm preparing or clearing
> up. Instead of puddings, I now have a piece of fruit half
> way between dinner and bedtime, and really look forward
> to it.

Taking Control

- Awareness brings you power. Write down as many endings as
  you can to the phrase: 'I overeat because . . .' Don't censor
  them, just write down anything that comes to mind, however
  far-fetched it may seem. It's a powerful step to get them all
  written down where you can see them more clearly. Then,
  take a look at your list of reasons and choose which ones you
  really want to keep using and which ones you want to
  discard. You might discover a different range of reasons
  by trying variations on this exercise: 'I eat junk food because .
  . .' 'I eat addictively because . . .'

- If you have difficulty figuring out what your justification is,
  just wait a while before eating until you know what it is. It
  doesn't matter how long this takes. The longer you wait, the
  clearer your justification will become. Sometimes you might
  blank out and go ahead and eat anyway. If this happens, you
  can figure out the reason you gave yourself afterwards.

- You can also notice justifications when you are buying items in the shops, ordering items from a menu and even when deciding which restaurant to visit. The choice to eat is often made at this time, even though you might actually eat the food later on.

- What works best is to identify the justifications you use most often. Then, either choose to use them or not. They may still occur to you from time to time but you can regard them as insufficient reasons to go ahead and eat.

- With a good enough justification you won't feel guilty, or at least not so guilty, about your addictive overeating. So challenging your justifications may not be easy; without them you no longer have 'good grounds' for feeding your addictive desire.

- Your biggest breakthroughs can happen during times of strong and difficult emotions. Clients tell me that they have learned to expect to feel their addictive desire to eat at these times, and, instead of satisfying it, they start to manage it, even in the middle of these feelings. The breakthrough occurs when they find out for themselves that the painful emotions – anger, sadness, rejection, for example – *didn't get any worse*. In fact, these feelings may even lighten up and pass more quickly through a rise in self-esteem from not overeating.

- If you call your overeating 'comfort eating' start to think of it as 'addictive eating'. Calling it comforting focuses on the perceived benefit only, which is how you justify it. It's more honest to call it addictive eating, which may bring some comfort as well as some unwelcome consequences later. Satisfying any addictive desire will often feel comforting, but not always – and it's usually at a cost.

- Your addictive thinking wants to keep all this hidden, so you may find it difficult at first. An addiction is always supported by lies, and when you've exposed a lie it's difficult to maintain. That's the point. The more you push yourself to do it, the easier it will become. Try not to judge yourself too harshly. Most people are addicted to something – caffeine, for example. Instead of condemning yourself, you could congratulate yourself for starting to do something about it – and appreciate yourself for all the things you're *not* addicted to!

Notes

1 For natural approaches to managing stress, anxiety and depression, read *Healing: Without Freud or Prozac* by Dr David Servan-Schreiber (Macmillan UK, 2003).

2 The Women's Nutritional Advisory Service has been providing help for women for over a decade and has an 85 per cent success rate in reducing symptoms of PMS. Nutritionist Maryon Stewart, who set up the service, has written a book called *No More PMS* (Vermilion, 1992).

3 Leslie Kenton, in *The New Ultrahealth* (Vermilion, 1995), refers to a number of different studies which support this, including the following: 'Dr Alexander Leaf, from Harvard Medical School, spent several years studying three cultures where the people were exceptionally long-lived . . . but who at the same time showed few signs of degenerative changes traditionally associated with age. They suffered neither tooth decay, heart disease, mental illness, obesity nor cancer . . . they led extremely active lives, regardless of their age, and had vigorous sex lives well into their eighties and nineties . . . They ate a very low-calorie diet. While the average Briton or American eats somewhere between 3,000 and 3,500 calories a day . . . they ate a mere 1,700 . . . low in fats and proteins from animal sources and high in fresh foods, a great many of them eaten raw . . . they had never heard of sugar.'

4 Overweight volunteers who claimed to be unable to lose weight, no matter what they ate, were studied at the Obesity Research Center at Columbia University. The researchers concluded: 'The failure of some obese subjects to lose weight while eating a diet they report as low in calories is due to an energy intake substantially higher than reported and an overestimation of physical activity . . . Whereas many people underreport their calorie intake, the degree of underreporting is greater in obese subjects.' *New England Journal of Medicine* 1992; 327:27 1893–1898.

And in *Nutritional Reviews* (1990; 48: 10, 373–379) '. . . considerable inaccuracy in self-reports of energy intake has been documented.'

5   'Energy balance only needs to be displaced by a tiny fraction for the cumulative effects to result in obesity. The fattest man in the world died recently in his mid-forties weighing 465 kg (73 stone). Even this enormous accumulation of fat required an excess equivalent to only a small bar of chocolate each day.' This is from Dr Andrew Prentice at the MRC Dunn Clinical Nutrition Centre, *British Medical Bulletin* 1997; 53,229-237, by permission of Oxford University Press.

6   A survey supported by the mental health charity Mind ('Food and Mood Project', June 2002) found an impressive 80 per cent had significant improvements in mood (including mood swings, depression and anxiety attacks) as a direct result of dietary changes. In some cases symptoms disappeared entirely. Vegetables, fruit, oily fish and water were found to be particularly helpful. Those foods which were found to have a negative effect were fried foods, sugar, caffeine, alcohol and chocolate.

   Healing: Without Freud or Prozac (Macmillan UK, 2003) contains a whole chapter with evidence regarding the link between depression and deficiencies in omega-3 fatty acids and folate (leafy greens).

7   One of the most thorough studies of eating disorders, conducted at the University of Minnesota with over 900 teenage girls, identified 'poor awareness of their feelings' as a key factor. 'These girls have trouble distinguishing among their most basic feelings. They may have a problem with their boyfriend, and not be sure whether they're angry, or anxious, or depressed – they just experience a diffuse emotional storm that they do not know how to deal with effectively. Instead they learn to make themselves feel better by eating; that can become a strongly entrenched emotional habit.' *Journal of Abnormal Psychology* (1993) 102(3):438–44.

8   A great deal of evidence indicates that by far the most effective treatment for depression is any form of physical exercise. Stronger self-esteem is also a major key, as is the development of optimism. As well as Branden's *The Six Pillars of Self-Esteem*, I recommend *How to Lift Depression Fast* by Joe Griffin and Ivan Tyrrell (HG Publishing, 2004).

9   '£11M lotto hulk binges to death' reported in the *Sun*, December 31 1996.

10   'An average 70-year-old person needs 500 fewer calories per day to
     maintain his or her body weight than an average 25-year-old. The
     average 80-year-old needs 600 fewer calories. In short, from around age
     20 onward, you need to take in about 100 calories per day less each
     decade to maintain the status quo.' From *Biomarkers: The Ten Keys to
     Prolonging Vitality* (Simon & Schuster, 1992).

11   'The increases in obesity seen in many Western countries over the past
     few decades, and the even larger increases in some of the Pacific
     Islanders whose countries have undergone dramatic lifestyle changes,
     are not reflections of genetic changes, but of gene expression facilitated
     by the environment. The most widely held view is that genes confer a
     susceptibility or predisposition to obesity and genetically predisposed
     individuals may be especially susceptible to aspects of lifestyle such as
     low activity and high fat diets, and gain weight more readily.' Reprinted
     by permission from *International Journal of Obesity*; 20, S1-S8 (1996)
     Macmillan Publishers Ltd.

CHAPTER 10

'My Body Made Me Do It'

In the middle of difficulty lies opportunity.
ALBERT EINSTEIN

Someone once explained their return to smoking by telling me that their body made them do it. I thought this was a delightful, albeit inaccurate, way to describe a common and central confusion around addictions. This is the fear that no matter how strong your intention to behave in new ways, your physically addicted body will compel you to act otherwise. Many of those who eat in addictive ways see their problem in these terms, believing that they get overwhelmed by physical cravings that compel them to eat.

There is a biochemical side to addiction. However, now that scientists have more clearly identified what goes on, it has become popular to think of addiction *purely* in terms of biochemistry, especially the chemistry of our 'control centre', the brain. This can be unhelpful. When we learn, for example, about how certain foods enhance the mood-altering neurotransmitter serotonin, it's easy to feel helpless when magical and mysterious chemicals seem to be running the show.

The reason this view is so widespread is that for

generations now, the scientific and medical community has readily acknowledged the effect the (physical) brain has on the (non-physical) mind, but absolutely refused to consider it a two-way communication. The notion that thoughts can alter the way the brain works has been regarded as unscientific because it cannot be easily explained. And yet, there's no scientific explanation of how the physical functions of the brain turn into thoughts. This is simply observed to be the case. And in recent years, thanks to modern brain-scanning technology, we have been able to observe that thoughts produce effects on the physical matter of the brain – *in ways that last*.

In this chapter we will look in more detail at how we direct our thoughts to create lasting, curative effects on the way the brain works with regard to addictive overeating. We won't be covering more techniques in this chapter but gaining greater understanding of what we've already looked at, especially in Chapters 5, 6 and 8.

As we've already seen, the feeling of craving, desire and attraction for food you don't need is activated by the conditioned response. What this means is that physical routes have been established in your brain – called neural pathways – that connect the cues with your desire for food. So, for example, you walk into the newsagent's shop and fancy a bar of chocolate. You're at the canteen for lunch and you want a pudding. You feel frustrated with the kids and reach for something sugary. You relax to watch television after dinner and feel like a snack.

Quite simply, you are reminded of food, and once the neural pathways have been established, the memory will be triggered *automatically*. It's essentially the same as any other memory but much exaggerated in an addiction. It becomes exaggerated because it's been reinforced many times but mostly through the influence of the 'reward chemicals' in the brain, especially dopamine. (1)

Whenever we feel pleasure and satisfaction, these reward chemicals have been released. They are what makes sex pleasurable and satisfying, so if you've ever thought to yourself that eating something was an orgasmic experience, you were absolutely right!

This is a survival mechanism at work. Way back when, if we came across a blackberry bush in the woods, it would support our survival to *enjoy* the berries and to *remember* where they were so that next year we could find our way back and get some more. Of course, part of our problem is that we live in such abundant times, given that we evolved to survive famine, not resist temptation. But it's also helpful to see that food manufacturers extract the most *enjoyable* and *memorable* components of food to sell to us. We keep buying them not because we need them but because they activate this reward system so effectively – in ways that are not unlike other addictive drugs such as cocaine and nicotine.

Any kind of food will activate the reward system to some extent, but fats and the high-GL carbs are more addictive because they magnify it. Dopamine in particular means that something is 'moreish' and is why, when you're experiencing addictive desire, you are likely to be wanting something with sugar and/or wheat and/or fat. (2)

Fats and high-GL carbs activate this motivational system so well that our desire for them has the strength and quality of a survival drive. Our most powerful means of survival is our brain, and when presented with addictive food it gets conned into thinking that our survival is at stake. So all of the brain's formidable processes are automatically brought into action, including the justifications and the denial. If you've ever been shocked by the devious mind games you can get into about food, just know that all of that conniving and bargaining is your brain trying to be very efficient at keeping you alive.

Once you've learned what kind of food is going to reward you the most, the dopamine starts to flood into your brain *just at the thought of eating it*. This flood of dopamine is your addictive desire, and it has the effect of motivating you towards that food, grabbing your attention and getting you lusting after it. This is the excitement of anticipation.

There's actually *more dopamine released in those moments of desire* than during eating, when you're satisfying the desire. This could be why the satisfaction of addictive desire can sometimes be a bit disappointing, when the experience of eating wasn't as exciting as you thought it was going to be. And why some people can at times feel compelled to eat even though they're sure they aren't going to enjoy the food (when they've already eaten too much, for example). And this is why the more intense feelings of addictive desire can create a kind of trance state, so that you feel 'possessed'.

The key is that neural pathways can be changed. Not only that, but unless they are changed you probably won't benefit in the long term.

The more often your addictive desire gets satisfied, the more familiar and established it gets, and the more it will reinforce and continue to trigger the reward pathways in the brain. Remember from Chapter 6 that the sight and smell of food can also be cues, and even photographs in advertisements and on television. Recovering cocaine addicts can get a craving triggered by the sight of talcum powder, long after detoxification. Remember too, from Chapter 8, that the process of eating often activates the addictive desire, so that you'll end meals wanting more.

The common view is that this feeling of addictive desire will force you to eat, so the only strategy is to avoid feeling it and to keep your mind on something else. The chances are you've already tried keeping yourself busy and changing your routines so that you don't encounter the cues in the first place. There may be times when you'll use an avoidance strategy – but know that it does not take you where you want to go. It will help you to understand why.

Changes That Last

The key is that neural pathways can be changed. Not only that, but unless they are changed you probably won't benefit in the long term. In fact, it has been proposed that *any* therapy works only to the extent that new neural pathways have been established. (3)

As for our goal of eating less, the time when you're working on these brain connections is *when you are feeling your unsatisfied addictive desire*. If you avoid the cue, nothing happens. You've successfully avoided feeling and feeding your addictive desire, but nothing has happened to alter the neural pathways, and so the conditioned response remains as potent as ever.

Strategies based on avoidance can only work up to a point, which is why the advice in this book is different from anything you've heard before. You take a massive leap forward when you understand that your addictive desire is your healing process. It's your healing process because *the mental effort you make to work through it* literally remoulds your brain by physically establishing new neural pathways.

You only get to do this when you're in the newsagent's shop, when you're in the canteen at lunch, when you're feeling angry with the kids, when you're watching television. Whether the desire is intense or fleeting, you focus on it and think yourself through it, as described in Chapter 6. It can be a real challenge at first – this is your withdrawal from addiction – but then it gets much easier *because the new pathways have been established.*

The effectiveness of this approach has only become apparent fairly recently, made possible through the fMRI and PET scans which enable us to see living, working brains with patterns of thought in action. What has been discovered through this technology is that the brain has the capacity to change itself. We now know that these neural connections aren't 'cast in stone' as was once thought and that we can deliberately intervene to forge new connections.

Research in many areas, such as obsessive-compulsive disorder, chronic depression, stroke rehabilitation, phobias, anxiety and panic attacks, demonstrates the power of directed thought to *permanently* alter the brain. These changes show up very clearly in the brain scans, along with reported improvements in behaviour and mood. The common element in recovery is deliberately paying attention to moments of difficulty and choosing new thoughts instead of passively following established neural pathways. (4)

This research points us towards these crucial elements:

■ It's your *conscious attention* that establishes new neural pathways, so it's essential to be aware of the addictive desire at the time it's happening.

▪ It's important to develop an *attitude of acceptance* towards the feeling of desire. This means not being upset by it, nor making it mean something else, such as signifying that you're greedy. The addictive desire is nothing more than an automatic memory, following a pathway that's already established in the brain.

▪ It will help you to make a distinction between this automatic reaction and *you* – your true self. *You* have the ability to observe that your brain is carrying a *false survival message*. This helps you to create some distance from your automatic, addictive thinking.

▪ And – most important of all – this process needs to be *self-directed* so it's essential to acknowledge your own free choice in the matter. You recognise that you're the one who's in charge; you determine how fast you take it, what moments of addictive desire you'll work through and what benefits you'll gain as a result. This is why.

Above Your Eyebrows

Your dopamine pathways run from the midbrain to an area called the prefrontal cortex. Situated towards the front of your forehead, the prefrontal cortex is the part of your brain where the real action takes place. This is the area you use when you turn your attention towards your addictive desire. As you think through your addictive desire, those brain cells become stronger, physically growing new connections. (5)

Brain scans show that it's the prefrontal cortex that

becomes active in the moments of making a decision for yourself. *It's not involved when subjects simply follow instructions.* (6)

And the prefrontal cortex is not used when we react mindlessly and automatically to an urge or impulse coming from the brain. How do we know that? Those unfortunate people who have had massive injury to this area, through an accident, prefrontal lobotomy or disease, don't have the capacity to control their own whims, and so their behaviour is chaotic and impulsive in inappropriate ways. They lose the ability to make decisions, to consider consequences of their actions and have no control over their emotions – simply because they are unable to use their prefrontal cortex.

The ability to control impulse is a very human capacity and is the last part of the brain to develop fully. If you've spent any time at all around an infant or toddler you know that we aren't born with it! This is why adults need to make so many choices on behalf of their children as much as they can, especially early on. (7)

Establishing new prefrontal cortex pathways could be a major challenge for you or a minor one, depending on where you start from. Ideally, this is a skill developed over the years of childhood, as parents and teachers patiently teach young ones how to make their own choices rather than simply follow orders. An upbringing that is far too strict, liberal or chaotic and unpredictable can hinder this process. *But it's never too late to start.* Adult brains can be remoulded too, and that's exactly what you're doing every time you work through your addictive desire to eat.

Brain scans show that it's the prefrontal cortex that becomes active in the moments of making a decision for yourself.

If you suspect that this will be a struggle for you, please keep in mind that when you do begin to connect with a genuine sense of choice more often, this will produce very exciting rewards in many areas of your life. And, at the very least, you will gain more control of your overeating.

This is what Chapter 5 is all about. At first, you might struggle with some of the symptoms of deprivation described in that chapter. As you repeatedly remind yourself that you've got choices, you'll find that your difficulties with deprivation evaporate. When you connect with that sense of choice, you'll know it has a very different feel to it, and it will be unmistakable when you've done it. Now you know why it makes such a huge difference: *you are accessing a different part of your brain.*

I know that some people have taken all this to mean that they should be, for example, 'choosing' chocolate ice cream instead of vanilla, or thinking in terms of 'making a choice' to eat croissants for lunch. It's essential to know that these can be chosen – otherwise there is no real choice to make – but progress only gets made through choices to accept the thoughts and feelings of desire for these addictive 'foods'. Then, *new neural connections become established with that addictive desire*. Then, you develop the ability not to eat ice cream or croissants – assuming that's what you want to achieve.

In the short term, you get control over your desires, impulses and attractions. But perhaps the most rewarding aspect of this process is that, as new prefrontal cortex connections are established, the dopamine pathways become less active. This means that your addictive desire begins to fade, becoming much less intense and much less persistent. (8)

This is ideally what we want to happen to our addictive memories: not to want the bar of chocolate when we walk into the newsagent's shop; not to want a pudding at lunch every day; not to want to eat every time we feel angry with the kids; not to be wanting food all evening, every evening. The first step is not to evade the thought of desire but to work through it. As prefrontal cortex connections are established, the desire diminishes. This is why, if you don't acknowledge choice, the desire persists and is even exaggerated, as we've seen in Chapters 6 and 8.

This is a completely natural process and it's entirely possible that you have already done it at times in the past. It's a process that's available to anyone with a prefrontal cortex! I'm just describing it so that you can use it in a more deliberate way. Your addictive desire is automatic; *your use of the prefrontal cortex in response is not*. Greater awareness of the deliberate effort that's needed gives you greater power.

You Call the Shots

If you ever think that developing impulse control sounds a bit dull, *just remember that you don't have to do it!* You don't have to do any of this, and you choose what desire to control and when. It's your life to create however you want. It's only a problem if *you* say it is, if your eating is controlled by addictive desire and you continually regret that. Do you really want to live your life feeling like a failure around food, and everything that means? The point is, you don't have to.

Most people don't acknowledge their freedom of choice, so it's inevitable that something else will be held responsible instead. Then, whatever that thing is, they regard themselves as victims of it. As victims they complain, 'It wasn't me – I didn't do it!' and explain, 'My body made me do it, my genes made me do it, my feelings made me do it, my parents made me do it, my partner made me do it, my culture made me do it, my job made me do it, my addiction made me do it.'

Then, instead of solving the problem, we get the perpetuation of the problem. It's so easy to blame our circumstances for our own reluctance to change, but the reality is that each one of us can choose to take control of our addictive overeating. We are only victims if we allow ourselves to be.

Your addictive desire is automatic and if you continue to live with it passively and unconsciously, nothing will change. By deliberate thinking you are refusing to accept that you are the victim of your biochemistry. *It's not your biochemistry that controls you, it's your belief that biochemistry controls you that undermines your ability to take control.* As Dr Schwartz says to his patients with obsessive-compulsive disorder, 'The brain's gonna do what the brain's gonna do, but you don't have to let it push you around.' (9)

Now you know why all those things you've tried before don't work; they've been ways to deny choice and avoid addictive desire. Now you know better. For example, if you eat addictively whenever you're bored, you've developed a conditioned response between boredom and addictive eating. So, it's fair to assume that the next time you feel bored, a release of dopamine means you'll want to eat. So, you allow yourself to feel bored just as much as you normally would. When you face your desire and don't try to fill the time in any other way, you work through it by making choices to change your priorities. You can only do that at the time it's happening, in those boring moments when you want to eat. You can't do it ahead of time.

If, after you've worked through your addictive desire, you then want to do something other than eat, by all means do that. If you're bored, a creative project can always be found. If you're feeling stressed, maybe a long, hot bath will help you to wind down. If you're feeling lonely, maybe a phone call will help. If you want to feel comforted, you can wrap yourself in a duvet and do nothing but appreciate yourself for all you've done recently.

The crucial element is that you don't attempt these things as a way to evade your addictive desire. First, you overcome your resistance, fear and conflict around the desire by looking it squarely in the face and making a clear choice about it. Then, you get on with your life.

IN OTHER WORDS: EMMA

Gillian's approach allowed me to prioritise my eating, not my weight. Before, I used to try to lose weight to look better, and I felt trapped, as though I was restricting my diet against my own will in order to be considered attractive by others. I would rebel against diets because I was angry that I 'had to lose weight' to feel good enough. Now, I find it very helpful to choose my eating habits for the sake of my health, energy and positivity. Those are things I can improve today. I can make healthy food choices from the moment I wake up, whereas I cannot wake up and decide to be a size 10 today. Weight is just the delayed result of my actions. Choosing what I ➤

eat is where my power is.

One of the most useful things about Gillian's technique is learning to see how I eat as an exercise in autonomous choice and chosen consequences. When I find myself standing in front of an open fridge, I now imagine myself as being like an atom that could move in one of several directions, mapping out a choice of pathways before me. A food choice represents taking a specific path, so I stop to think where it will lead me. I try to look beyond the moment to see which choice will leave me feeling better later on. I know that if I choose foods that will nourish me, or simply if I choose not to eat when I do not need to, I will end up going to bed that night more relaxed and hopeful about the next day, without the churning anxiety and physical discomfort that follow, for instance, a sugar binge. Food has a real effect on my mood, and, sadly, eating fruit or vegetables will leave me calmer and more confident than eating chocolate, which tastes great, but has no benefit beyond the two seconds of chewing a mouthful.

It has been enormously helpful to learn to recognise my addictive desire to eat for what it is. This desire can feel like a series of little electric shocks which build until I am impelled to stand up and get food. Gillian's technique made me realise that the desire itself does not hurt me. When I experience the addictive desire I am not actually in pain, and if I sit it out there will be a much bigger payoff than if I eat every time I am bored or stressed. I still haven't mastered sitting with the addictive desire every time it occurs, but at least I now ➤

> know the task at hand. When the addictive desire strikes,
> I now tell myself that so long as it is there and I have not
> acted on it, I am safe. My anxiety tells me to silence the
> nagging desire by eating, but I now recognise that I can
> acknowledge it, coexist with it and get on with my life.
>
> This didn't work until I actually started doing it. I read
> Gillian's book, thought 'yes, this is great' but mastering
> the theory wasn't enough. In order to get the changes I
> want, I need to put the ideas into practice at the moments
> when I am actually experiencing the addictive desire to eat.

Taking Control

- Be willing to be repetitive. It's very much like advertising,
  where nobody brings a slogan or brand name into the world
  with a single announcement. The ad is repeated over and
  over again; that's what makes it become a household name.
  In the same way, it's not just a matter of reading this book
  and understanding the theory. What makes the difference is
  launching your own advertising campaign to promote these
  ideas in your everyday thoughts, so that in time it becomes
  your familiar way of thinking.

- Owning choice makes all the difference. The most intense,
  difficult and persistent cravings are symptoms of deprivation
  created through the denial of choice. This denial of choice is
  usually associated with an obsession with weight loss, years
  of dieting, prohibitive thinking (in general) and lower levels
  of self-esteem.

- Just like emotions such as anger and sadness, addictive desire can be conjured up at will. That's what actors do when they deliberately create genuine feelings by accessing memories associated with a particular emotion. You can do the same with your feeling of addictive desire, just to practise managing it. This means you encourage feelings of temptation so that you can face and work through them. As an example, whenever I'm in a deli, I often go right up to the glass case with the pastries and take a good look at them, taking a brief moment to connect with my desire and my choices.

- It really helps to remember the reward pathways in those moments of desire. Your addictive desire is nothing other than an established brain connection with a certain cue; it doesn't matter if you can't identify the cue, as they can sometimes be quite subtle. If the idea of growing new neural connections seems daunting, just know that you do this *any time you learn anything*.

- Conditioned responses to emotions are more difficult to dissolve. This means that your addictive desire triggered by feelings such as anger and frustration is likely to be more persistent. In time, though, it too will fade. It will make a big difference to accept it when it's there and to remember it's just another conditioned response in the brain.

NOTES

1 Whenever a reward is involved, the connections that form neural pathways are bonded more strongly. As well as dopamine, a number of other reward chemicals, such as beta-endorphins and serotonin, are part of this reaction. *Physiology & Behavior* (2002) 76; 389–395.

2 Our preference for fats and sweets is thought to be inherent; not so long ago we simply would not have encountered as much of them as we do today. When we eat the high-GL carbs our bodies get a surge of glucose and adrenaline, so it's probably this stimulant effect that strengthens those dopamine pathways.

 However, there are also cultural and personal responses to food. Paul Rozin at the University of Pennsylvania has done much research that questions biochemistry as the only, or even the primary, factor in our food preferences.

3 'All forms of psychotherapy – from psychoanalysis to behavioral interventions – are successful to the extent to which they enhance change in relevant neural circuits.' From *The Neuroscience of Psychotherapy* (Norton, 2002) by Louis Cozolino, PhD, professor of psychology at Pepperdine University.

4 'The wilful focusing of attention is not only a psychological intervention. It is also a biological one. Through changes in the way we focus attention, we have the capacity to make choices about what mental direction we will take; more than that, we also change, in scientifically demonstrable ways, the systemic functioning of neural circuitry.' From *The Mind and the Brain* by Jeffrey M. Schwartz MD and Sharon Begley (HarperCollins, 2002). Examples of this kind of research can also be found in: *A User's Guide to the Brain* (Little, Brown & Co, 2001) by John J. Ratey, MD, Associate Clinical Professor of Psychiatry at Harvard Medical School, and, if you prefer a lighter read, in my book, *Willpower!* (Vermilion, 2003).

5 'Given the strong evidence for the involvement of the prefrontal cortex in

the wilful selection of self-initiated responses, the importance of knowing we can modulate the brain activity in that very area with a healthy dose of mindfulness can't be overstated.' From *The Mind and the Brain* by Jeffrey M. Schwartz MD and Sharon Begley (HarperCollins, 2002).

6   Brain scans were compared for two different tasks. In one, subjects were told to speak a particular word or move a specified finger. Brain activity was compared with another task where subjects decided for themselves which word to speak or which finger to move. The prefrontal areas were only active when subjects made conscious decisions about their actions. 'Towards a Functional Anatomy of Volition', *The Volitional Brain, Journal of Consciousness Studies* 6, 8–9, (1999).

7   'The prefrontal cortex performs the "executive functions" of the brain – the ability to regulate emotion, anticipate and plan for the future, make rational decisions and shape behaviour towards attainment of motivational goals. Psychological development, in neuroscience terms, is maturation of the prefrontal cortex.' *The Mind-Brain Relationship* by Regina Pally (Karnac, 2001).

8   Research has demonstrated that Pavlovian conditioning can be 'extinguished' by experiencing the cue (e.g. walking into your kitchen) without the conditioned reinforcement (e.g. snacking). This process of 'extinction' (the fading of addictive desire) takes place in the prefrontal cortex. There are a number of studies on this; a key paper can be found in the science journal *Nature* (M. R. Milad, G. J. Quirk. 2002;420(6911): 70–4).

9   From *The Mind and the Brain* by Jeffrey M. Schwartz MD and Sharon Begley (HarperCollins, 2002).

CHAPTER 11

Addiction and Self-esteem

There is perhaps no psychological skill more fundamental than resisting impulse.
DANIEL GOLEMAN, EMOTIONAL INTELLIGENCE

Now that we have explored the main psychological aspects, let's take a closer look at the relationship between addictive eating and self-esteem. To me, this is crucial because it's nothing other than the exhilaration of stronger self-esteem that keeps me going when the going gets tough. In fact, I think it only ever got tough at times when I'd forgotten just how much my eating affects my self-esteem.

For self-esteem read happiness. It's what I feel when I wake up in the morning glad to be who I am, eager to tackle my day. It's easy to assume this depends on external circumstances – but have you noticed that your spirits can rise even though circumstances haven't changed in any significant way? Next time it happens, see if it could be that you recently reinforced one of the 'six pillars' of your self-esteem, as described in Chapter 4. Maybe you asserted yourself in a new way, you owned your choices about something or you became more purposeful about getting something done. That's self-esteem in action.

A great many people aren't aware of these shifts – especially if they have been encouraged to think of their self-esteem primarily in terms of outward signs of success, status, achievement and/or appearance, which, unfortunately, is often the case. As Dr Branden says, 'The tragedy of many people's lives is that they look for self-esteem in every direction except within, and so they fail in their search.' (1)

When it comes to taking control of addictive eating, fully engaging with genuine, private self-esteem as your motivation is a major change to make. It's entirely possible you haven't made this change yet, and appearance is still your priority in your choices about food. Our culture encourages this so it's not surprising, and it's likely you will be tempted down some false paths as a result.

Avoidance Strategies

One false path is found in substituting other behaviours. They are often addictions themselves and in many cases don't contain a lot of calories: cigarettes, chewing gum, diet sodas, diet foods, coffee, tea, alcohol, and excessive shopping, work and/or exercise. They might help you to keep your weight down, but they don't contribute to stronger self-esteem. Any addictive behaviour will erode your self-esteem, and too much caffeine, tobacco, artificial sweeteners and/or alcohol can be as damaging to your health as overeating. Not only that, but they won't help you to overcome your addictive relationship with food either. (2)

When weight loss is your primary goal, these kinds of avoidance and substitution strategies might make sense in the short term. There's no end of things you can do instead of eating, but trying to control your eating through them simply doesn't work in the longer term. You will achieve only a partial, conditional resolution of your addictive desire to eat and therefore gain only a partial – and temporary – success.

This is especially true of smoking as a way to control eating because it tends to destroy health and self-esteem to such a degree. And smoking often satisfies your addictive desire to eat, so if you are a smoker, it's only when you've quit that you will be able to deal properly with your addiction to food. If you are an ex-smoker, be aware that your desire to smoke may surface when you cut back on your addictive eating, especially if you gained weight when you stopped smoking. This indicates that you substituted food for cigarettes, so your desire to smoke and your desire to eat will be interchangeable. (3)

Another false path is the use of pharmaceuticals designed to reduce your addictive appetite, such as 'fen/phen', which became extremely popular in the United States a number of years ago. People who took these appetite-suppressant drugs lost interest in overeating, feeling satisfied with a lot less food. Their addictive desire had been taken away, at least in part.

Although this may sound like the miracle cure we all have been waiting for, this is a long way from the truth. 'Fen/phen' was withdrawn from the market due to dangerous side-effects, especially damage to the heart. But before its danger became obvious, the drug was officially approved, promoted in the media as 'the most important weight-loss discovery of the century' and prescribed to thousands.

It has been widely recognised that its approval was

premature, having been pushed through the process by the hugely influential pharmaceutical industry. Do you think anything has changed since then? The pharmaceutical companies are still working hard to develop a 'miracle diet pill' which will hit the jackpot for them, but unknown factors are inevitable when products first come on to the market. (4)

All pharmaceuticals are potentially dangerous. In very extreme cases the danger can be worth the risk, but when it comes to weight loss that's not the most common consideration. Any pharmaceutical solution to overeating would need to be taken for life because there can never be a permanent 'cure'. Using a pharmaceutical temporarily would be like going on a shopping spree with a credit card; you pay the bill later on but you still end up paying. But the real concern is that the medication could actually make things worse in the longer term. (5)

The next generation of 'anti-obesity' medications are known as 'anti-craving agents' and damp down addictive appetite through their influence on neurotransmitters. The one that's received the most media attention so far is called rimonabant (trade name Accomplia). However, the blocking of neurotransmitters isn't limited just to the desire for food, and its efficacy and safety over the long term is questionable. (6)

Whenever a new pharmaceutical aimed at tackling overeating comes on to the market, consider whether the medication is to be taken for life, and if not, what happens when the medication is stopped? Do people simply return to overeating and is their problem made worse? Consider what might happen if you ever need to stop taking the medication, for any reason.

This is where you can see why it's such a false path to have weight loss as your primary goal. So many people assume that all they really need to do is to *lose the weight*. If only they could do that, then they would eat sensibly, have greater self-esteem and everything would be fine. They think that with the weight lost they would be starting off with a clean slate – ignoring the fact that nothing has changed about their potential for addictive overeating. This is why weight-loss quick-fixes such as the Atkins Diet and pharmaceuticals hold such incredible allure, but this is also why they don't work long term. In order to achieve *lasting* weight loss, that whole line of thinking needs to be turned around.

Life's Too Short!

I know it can be difficult not to make appearance your main priority, but the more you think in terms of fat and thin, the more you are missing the boat. *I want to suggest that you will not lose weight – and keep it off – until you don't care about it as much as you care about your health and your self-esteem.*

It makes a profound difference to prioritise your health and self-esteem instead of setting out to improve your appearance. As an example, if you feel like eating before your Time (see page 105), this doesn't necessarily affect what you look like. You are unlikely to gain weight if

> **So many people assume that all they really need to do is to lose the weight.**

you eat lunch at 12.45 instead of 1pm. When you care about your self-esteem, you wait until 1pm simply because you said you would, which strengthens the power of your word to yourself. And this regard for and development of self-discipline is exactly what you need in order to continue.

When appearance is your priority, you're likely to make trade-offs such as justifying overeating by promising yourself a longer session in the gym later that day. There's little in this kind of decision that supports your health and self-esteem; it's all about appearance. It's about wanting to overeat as much as you can get away with and still look okay.

You'll know that you haven't yet made this genuine change in motivation because you will continue to yo-yo diet. You might yo-yo just a bit, losing and regaining very modest amounts of weight each time. Or you might yo-yo a great deal, reaching your goal weight each time and then regaining the weight lost. This is far more dangerous to your health than just staying at the heavier weight. And (in case you don't know!) it's also a bit of a nightmare to live with. (7)

When your goal is genuine self-esteem you make health your priority. Weight loss will follow – and is much more likely to last. What helps the most in making this shift in motivation is experiencing the stronger self-esteem which comes from eating less.

You will never gain self-esteem from eating addictively because, by definition, it's bad for your health. The typical denial of addictive thinking means that you probably don't fully acknowledge the cost to your health, and it's easy to do that because the effects tend to be so very gradual.

Just as one cigarette doesn't give a smoker lung cancer, one chocolate biscuit won't make you diabetic, create a cancerous tumour or block your arteries. But smokers don't smoke just one cigarette and overeaters don't eat just one tiny scrap of trans fat or the occasional morsel of highly processed carbohydrate. When you eat addictively, possibly every day, these effects add up – even though you hardly notice them at the time.

Many people like to hold on to the philosophy that 'life is for living – so eat, drink and be merry!' Recently someone explained this outlook to me, dismissing my regard for a healthy lifestyle. They aim to live life to the full, they said, to enjoy all of their indulgences right up to the end, with no regrets about a body that's been thoroughly used up and totally worn out.

If our health is all down to luck, this could make sense. Luck certainly plays a part, as do our genes, but the main contribution has to do with life-long lifestyle choices about diet, smoking, alcohol and exercise. Of course it's inspiring to live life to the full, and I don't think I'd say no to the occasional indulgence, whatever my age. But I prefer to be able to see whatever it is I'm indulging in, not to have my hands crippled with arthritis or paralysed by strokes so that I can pick it up myself, and not to be in chemotherapy treatment so that I'm able to enjoy it as well. I can't say for sure that I'll pull that off for the rest of my life – but I aim to try my best.

The truth is that our bodies don't become used up and worn out through living life to the full. Our bodies become filled with pain and disease through a lifetime of addictive abuse coupled with plain old ignorance about good nutrition. I don't believe that someone who has struggled through their last decade or so with the poor health that addictive eating brought them is likely to say, at the end of their life, 'If only I'd eaten more!' (8)

When you think about it, could it be that your 'life is for living' philosophy is nothing but another justification for your addictive eating? At some point most people get 'wake-up calls' that cause them to question it. A wake-up call may arrive in the news that someone their age just had a stroke.

Or they are diagnosed as diabetic or as having high blood pressure. Or they get cancer or something that might be cancer. Then many, although by no means all, will drop the 'life is for living' philosophy and realise that life is for *living!* Then they start to make big changes in the way they eat, discovering willpower they never knew they had.

The truth is that our bodies don't become used up and worn out through living life to the full. Our bodies become filled with pain and disease through a lifetime of addictive abuse coupled with plain old ignorance about good nutrition.

So why not pay closer attention to the wake-up calls and be more willing to act on them before they get too loud? Prevention is *infinitely* better than cure – and you don't need to become obsessive about it. It's only your addiction that's going to object. You can find your very own, personal wake-up calls in any symptoms of poor health or low energy you may have, and in your own experience of lower self-esteem.

Acting the Part

Strong self-esteem isn't a luxury, it's a necessity. When it's missing we are more likely to experience periods of boredom, anxiety, sadness and even despair. We may try to avoid these feelings with a busy schedule but will increasingly seek to comfort – or numb – ourselves in addictions such as overeating until we experience very little pleasure without them. But this only makes the problem worse by further undermining our self-esteem. This causes us to find less and less pleasure in ourselves, and leaves us more likely to turn to addictions in an attempt to bring relief from our fundamental dislike of ourselves.

This vicious circle is most noticeable when we are on our own. With nobody to distract us or assure us of our worth, we are exposed to our own dissatisfaction with ourselves. This is partly why so many people eat addictively most often when they are alone. They don't want others to see how much they eat anyway, because other people's approval of them is always more important than their own.

The solution is self-esteem, which is strengthened by an increased sense of self-worth combined with a sense of competence at living. Both of these aspects are undermined when you overeat. This might seem to be confirmed when you look in the mirror, but it's the loss of control over food that erodes your self-esteem and that in turn makes a major contribution to depression. The time you actually spend eating, when you're feeling comforted and rewarded, provides relief. But you know that's very temporary and followed by regret, guilt and more depression later on. By managing addictive desire you will begin to restore a sense of self-worth *and* competence – which contributes in no small way to lifting any depression.

If you can see even some relevance here to your situation, the only step you need to take is to connect to this in those moments of desire. You recall the improvement in your life you'll gain if you don't satisfy that desire. That's the crucial mental effort required to make a real, lasting change.

The tragedy of low self-esteem is believing you're not valuable enough to stop overeating. Who wouldn't get depressed about that? Any symptoms of poor health you may have, together with our extreme cultural judgement of excess fat, simply serve to confirm it. If you find you cannot care enough about yourself to start to do things differently, at least you can 'fake it till you make it'. Act as if your life is precious. Pretend to honour yourself more, act accordingly – and the stronger self-esteem will follow.

Acting accordingly means using what you've learned in this book to strengthen the 'six pillars' (see Chapter 4) of your self-esteem:

1   You live more consciously by becoming aware of your addictive desire to eat food you don't need and the ways in which you try to justify satisfying that desire.

2   You gain self-acceptance as you start to eat in a way that honours your worth by supporting your health. You become more self-accepting when you accept that your addictive desire to eat is an inevitable memory of past overeating rather than the sign that you are flawed, greedy and/or self-destructive. Then, instead of resigning yourself to a life of uncontrollable overeating, you can gain acceptance of your unsatisfied desire, at least sometimes.

3   You gain self-responsibility whenever you remind yourself that it's your choice whether or not you satisfy your addictive desire: you always have the freedom to eat anything you want, and as much as you want.

4   You practise self-assertion when you say 'no thanks' to others, both in refusing food when it's appropriate and in refusing to prioritise looking a certain way in order to gain their approval.

5   You live purposefully by consciously declaring your physical and emotional health as your primary goal, and set out – choice by choice – to achieve that goal.

6   You have integrity when you keep your word to yourself

by sticking to your intentions – Times and Plans, for example – and when you spot the lies you tell yourself about what and how much you eat.

New Signs of Success

Perhaps all this sounds like far too much to remember. All you need to *do* is switch your focus from how much you weigh to whether or not you are working through your addictive desire to eat. As with any goal, it's important to be able to check on how you're doing as you go along. Instead of seeing success solely in terms of getting into smaller size clothes, start to create new standards of success:

▪ *Choosing Times and Plans, and keeping to them* (see pages 105–9). This brings you a real sense of control.
▪ *A more positive response to addictive desire.* This is a sign you have shifted your motivation from weight loss to taking control. When weight is all you care about, there's no reason to accept the uncomfortable feeling of an unsatisfied addictive desire; you could avoid it and get the same result. When dealing with addiction is your aim, it makes perfect sense because this is exactly where your success lies. And you get to lose weight too!
▪ *A more positive response to natural hunger.* As a result you have more energy and feel lighter in your body instead of heavy from overeating. This is a sign you have worked through your addictive thinking, and no longer feel deprived when you eat less.
▪ *Better health and vitality.* This comes from eating less and making healthier choices about what you do eat.

■ *Eating more of your food earlier in the day and less in the evenings.* Most addictive overeating is done in the evening. This means you digest food when you are the least active, which is not good for your health. It's only when you have come to terms with your addictive appetite, which usually surfaces later in the day, that you can start to correct the balance. (9)

■ *Staying off the scales.* This means you are developing your sense of self-worth based on your opinions of you, not on what other people see.

■ *Keeping this process and any weight loss as private as possible.* This means you are doing this more for yourself, because you like being in control of your eating. Taking control of overeating is a profound change in the way you live and in what your values are. When you discover that you can cope with life's ups and downs without overeating, this will mean far more to you than anything anybody else can ever say.

IN OTHER WORDS: JENNIFER

Before I found this approach, my life had always been full of stress, difficulty and a wrongness that I can't even put into words. I didn't understand why I couldn't live like other people, why I always had problems, why I never felt okay. For most of my life I had struggled with food and had developed an addiction to it. This was so severe that at one time I hardly came out of the house for a year and felt so depressed and out of control that I constantly thought about suicide. Despite all of this, I managed to ➤

finish my degree, producing a dissertation on eating disorders which got me on to a PhD course doing the same. Obviously this did make a big difference to my life but, despite all this, my problems were still there. I felt bad inside and very out of control around food, frequently alternating between bingeing and trying to diet to lose weight.

Worst of all were the days when I binged, which was often. I would wake up in the middle of the night, anxious and shaky from all the insulin my huge carbohydrate intake had induced, bloated, distressed and terribly scared at what I had done. And then, for the next few days, I'd be depressed, full of despair and suffering from insomnia. I was also beginning to develop problems with my health such as acne, frequent cystitis and a constant cold.

As soon as I started to read Eating Less, for the first time ever I had hope. I knew straight away that this book was going to make a difference to my life. I couldn't believe how well Gillian understood my problems, like no one ever before and even better than I had ever understood them myself. I gained comfort, balance and control from using Times and Plans, and I can't describe the liberation and empowerment I experienced by remaining aware that, instead of surrendering to my addictive desire to eat, I could choose to accept it instead.

Now, I don't have massive, self-destructive binges any more. I am able to buy food for the week and still have enough left by the end of it. Before, anything remotely edible in my house would have been consumed within a ➤

day or so of when it got there. I now feel relaxed and free around food. It changed my life to discover that I didn't need to be perfect and that I had free choice. But most of all, through this and through overcoming my addiction, I discovered how to raise my self-esteem.

Raising my self-esteem has been the answer I'd long been looking for. It has made everything feel right at last, reducing my previous mass of overwhelming problems to simple, normal, everyday concerns. It's what has changed the anxiety and depression which filled my life into frequent laughter, happiness and simple enjoyment of living. I could not possibly detail all the ways in which this book has made such a difference, but these teachings have created a shift in my thinking, and thus also my actions, which has finally enabled me to be the person I was supposed to be. Being in control of food now is just the beginning.

Taking Control

- Maintaining a real sense of choice is crucial in dealing with addictive eating, and strengthens your self-esteem as well. You are most likely to forget about choice *after* having over-eaten. This is the most important time to reconnect by thinking, 'I can eat like that, I can continue to eat like that, and I never have to make any changes at all.' Recall the whole picture of the choices open to you, including the undesired consequences of overeating and the alternative of managing addictive desire.

- What might you be doing in order to avoid feeling your

addictive desire to eat? Smoking, shopping or keeping yourself extra busy? Make a plan to deal with this so that you can gain a more complete acceptance of your addictive desire. This is how you make real, lasting changes in your relationship with food.

- If you are someone whose self-esteem tends to be fragile, be especially careful during those times when your esteem feels particularly low. This is when you are more vulnerable to addictive eating, not so much because you are overwhelmed by intolerable emotions – the common myth – but because *you've lost sight of your worth*. At these times you can begin to restore your esteem by taking control of one thing you can control: what you eat. So, you can either act out and reinforce your feelings of worthlessness by overeating, or start to act as if you deserve better.

- Find out what diseases members of your family have suffered or died from. This will give you clues to your genetic inheritance, and therefore what you are likely to be susceptible to. Find out how food affects these conditions and this will show you which foods could be especially dangerous for your health. Remember you will still have the choice to eat them. You will still experience a desire for them. And you will probably try to justify eating them.

  This applies just as much if members of your family have died as a result of addiction – to smoking, drinking or eating, for example. This indicates that you might have a genetic predisposition to addiction, so the techniques and principles in this book will be even more valuable for you.

Notes

1   From *The Six Pillars of Self-Esteem* by Nathaniel Branden, PhD (Bantam, 1994).

2   A study by University College London (not yet published) has followed 3,000 children aged 11 to 16 and found *no weight difference* between those who smoke and those who do not. Nicotine does raise the metabolic rate and suppress appetite, but the body quickly adapts so that smokers are very soon no better off.

3   Whether you are a smoker or an ex-smoker, my book *How To Stop Smoking And Stay Stopped For Good* (Vermilion, 1992) will show you how to deal with your addictive desire to smoke, without substituting food.

4   The *New England Journal of Medicine* (28 August, 1997) published an editorial on diet pills which included the following: 'It has never been shown, and it is highly implausible, that appetite-suppressant drugs can maintain weight loss indefinitely. To date, studies of these drugs have demonstrated efficacy only for short-term weight loss. Their safety if taken over a period of many years is doubtful, since the risk of serious toxicity appears to increase with the duration of use.'

A paper published in the *Journal of the American Medical Association* (2002; 287: 2215–2220) reviewed the problem of 'adverse drug reactions' to prescription medications in general and concluded: 'Serious adverse drug reactions commonly emerge after Food and Drug Administration approval. The safety of new agents cannot be known with certainty until a drug has been on the market for many years.'

5   According to an article on appetite suppressants in *Time* magazine (23 September, 1996), as soon as people stopped taking 'fen/phen' their serotonin levels dropped dramatically and remained low for many weeks. It is even thought that the serotonin receptors may have been permanently damaged and never returned to normal.

6   An article about rimonabant in the *Guardian,* 'Can taking a pill really help

you to lose weight and stop smoking?' (2 September, 2004) questions the wisdom of a drug that alters normal mental processes, is intended for permanent use, and could impair motivation in all areas of life, including relationships and the workplace. Another *Guardian* article (10 January, 2005) reported side-effects during the rimonabant trials of increased irritability, depression and anxiety. These faded in the second year of use, but so did the weight loss! Rimonabant led to an average loss of 5kg over one year, but no more weight was lost in the second year. When the medication was stopped, subjects returned to their original weight.

7   See Reference 2 in Chapter 2.

8   The two main causes of blindness are both connected to poor nutrition. It's a common complication of diabetes, and many develop blindness through macular degeneration, associated with oxidative stress. There is no cure for either, so the best strategy is prevention by eating lower-GL carbs and plenty of antioxidant foods. In other words, mostly vegetables, whole grains and some fruit, which will help a great deal with arthritis and strokes as well.

9   Some people find it helpful to have a small snack at bedtime as it can help to balance blood sugar levels and help them get to sleep and sleep right through the night. However, it's not a good idea to sleep on a full stomach, trying to digest a whole meal while you are inactive, horizontal and when your digestive system has slowed down. Even more important, the work of repairing and rebuilding lean mass goes on at night aided by growth hormones, and these are greatly impaired when there are digestive hormones in the bloodstream.

CHAPTER 12

Failing with Style

Freedom is not worth having if it does not include the freedom to make mistakes.
MAHATMA GANDHI

I don't know of anyone (including myself!) who has consistently used this approach to take control of their eating, with each and every encounter with food. I doubt that there's anyone who hasn't blown it at some point, made mistakes, overeaten and later regretted it. Some have lost the plot completely, and forgotten whole chunks of this technique. I hope you can see that it's perfectly reasonable to be on a learning curve, and that it's inevitable there will be ups and downs along the way. But what this really means is that at times *you will fail*.

Of all the challenges you'll meet in your efforts to eat less, the most difficult could be in facing up to the inevitability of some failure. However, there's failure and there's failure. There's losing control and giving up entirely on the whole idea. And there's *failing with style*, which is what this chapter is all about.

Mistakes are not the problem. The problem is believing they should never happen. What makes the difference is making fewer and fewer mistakes as you go along. And any time you have seriously lost your way, what makes the difference is knowing how to get back on track. In fact, not only is failure inevitable but to some extent *it's highly recommended!*

Being Imperfect

If you tend to be a bit of a perfectionist, it will help you enormously to give up any ideas you have of eating in a perfect way. Nobody can pull that off for the rest of their lives.

First of all, there is no such thing as an absolute definition of addictive eating, and there never can be. You can only say whether or not you eat addictively in terms of degree: either 'a great deal' or 'not very much' or somewhere in between. Taking control of overeating is, by its very nature, imperfect.

Aspiring to perfection will get in your way. If you think perfection is a reasonable goal, then no matter what you accomplish you'll focus on the one thing that's wrong, and everything gets cancelled out and becomes meaningless. Perfectionism sets up an 'all or nothing' attitude, where your eating is either perfect or perfectly dreadful. Living like this is like being on a roller-coaster ride, flying high one day and crashing down the next.

> **Mistakes are not the problem. The problem is believing they should never happen.**

It may well be that perfectionism was the only way you have been able to get any sense of control over your eating in the past. Whether following a diet, abstaining from particular foods or doing your version of not eating rubbish, *you had to do it perfectly or not at all*. But then, any time it's not perfect, you don't have anything else to use.

Perfectionism may attract you because you think it will bring you security; that if you use the technique perfectly, you'll be sure to stay in control. But the truth is that you could use these techniques absolutely to the letter for any period of time, and then start to do a lot of overeating, completely out of control. Why? Because it's not perfection that leads you to succeed in the long term; *it's gaining the ability to manage your addictive desire to eat*. When you have achieved that to a significant extent, then, even when you do eat addictively, you can get back into control by starting to deal with your addictive desire.

This is often something I hear from people who have done one of my courses. They tell me that when they 'blow it' they don't give up entirely as they used to, but get right back into eating in the way they really want. They are able to do this because they know how to work through their addictive desire – when in the past all they could do was follow some particular guidelines, whatever they were.

If you are a perfectionist when it comes to eating, I strongly urge you to make deliberate mistakes. Whenever you notice that you are in your 'perfect mode' go ahead and eat in a way that breaks that state of perfection. This could mean eating a type of food that you would only ever eat when you're bingeing and out of control. Sugar buns, perhaps. Or it could be eating spontaneously sometimes, before your Time or after your Plan. Aim to screw it up 10 or 20 per cent of the time, or whatever percentage works for you.

The 'perfect mode' can be exhilarating, so you will need to be willing to give up some of that. The benefit is that you smooth out the roller-coaster ride of 'out of control' and 'in control' eating, so that it's more like a bumpy road. When your 'out of control' eating is not so different from your 'in control' eating, you will feel much more relaxed and confident about the whole business. This confidence is something I hear about from clients, even a long time after they've done my course. *No one* follows the technique perfectly, but in general they eat healthier food, and less of it.

Please note that if you don't have a tendency towards perfectionism, you won't need to build in a 'screw-up' rate, because you will do that naturally. Some people will take on this approach in a far from perfect, even half-hearted way. If this is your style, it won't help you to use 'making mistakes' as a justification for even more overeating.

For just about everybody, though, making mistakes can get out of hand at times. At these times it will be a good idea to return to the sections detailed below, which give you the signposts you'll need to get back to a greater sense of control.

Getting Back on Track

At the end of Chapter 1 we looked at the three factors that determine whether or not you have control of addictive overeating. *All three* are an essential part of the process, and you'll find that it won't hold together if one is missing. Although we've looked at each one separately, they are very much interrelated. So, when you've really lost the plot, just take a good look at these three factors.

You will need to think carefully about them, though. I've had a number of conversations with clients who weren't doing so well later on, where they said something like, 'I understand all of what you are teaching, but I'm just not using it.' When we talk a bit, though, I always find there's something significant that they are not understanding at all. So it's clear to me, having worked on this for many years, that what this is about is keeping yourself open to the possibility of learning more.

Here's a summary of the issues and what chapters to review:

What's Your Motivation?

In Chapters 2, 3 and 4 we looked at the questions:

- Why do you eat or not eat something?
- If you want to change anything about your eating, why do you want to do that?

It's entirely possible that your appearance will dominate your motivation for any number of reasons. Perhaps because you've lost weight or because you haven't, or because a friend has lost more weight than you or because you're going to be 'on show' in some way. You know from this book, even if you didn't know before, that what works best in the long term is to prioritise your health. But you live in a culture that tells you otherwise. Your friends may tell you otherwise, as will the media and maybe your family. Everybody tells you, in all kinds of direct or subtle ways, that what matters is appearance, and it takes some awareness in order to stand your ground on this issue.

Health and weight don't necessarily go hand in hand. If you saw the brilliant documentary *Super Size Me* you'll have seen filmmaker Morgan Spurlock eating everything (breakfast, lunch and dinner) at McDonald's for one month. After three weeks he was depressed, lethargic, addicted, and his blood tests so alarming that his doctors urged him to abandon the project. This is an extreme example, of course, but my point is that he wasn't over his healthy weight range and still looked pretty good!

When you fall back into seeing success and failure primarily, or even exclusively, in terms of weight, you're likely to lose control of your eating. If you experience big variations in both the quality and quantity of what you eat – if you are bingeing on junk food one day and nibbling on celery the next – this is usually because weight loss is a primary goal. What's happening is that whenever you think about eating or not eating something, your weight, shape and size are all that really matter.

Your preoccupation with appearance will blind you to the more private and personal rewards of taking control. *While you are out of control, though, one thing you can discover is that being in control of your eating has greater value to you than only losing weight.* Keep observing the difference in the quality of your life in any way other than your appearance. Chapters 4 and 7 will help you to identify this far more effective kind of motivation. (1)

Are You Remembering it's Your Choice?

It's possible that things will go well at first, at least partly because you are 'being good'. In other words, you're complying with a new set of instructions – Times, Plans, managing desire and eating healthy food – in the same way you have complied with diets or abstinence in the past.

Although compliance brings success for a while, it doesn't work long term, as we saw in Chapters 5 and 10.

At first it can be difficult to know whether or not you're complying. If you are, all that will happen is that at some point you'll start to rebel – and that's when you can start to make progress. At this point you'll begin to feel deprived, feel stronger addictive desire and/or begin to eat more addictively, probably latching on to some compelling justification you've just discovered.

Remember that a fear usually drives the reluctance to embrace freedom of choice: that giving yourself permission to overeat will lead to even more eating. The automatic reaction is to deny choice in order to eat less. Watch out for prohibitive and authoritarian thoughts, such as 'I mustn't eat any more!' and 'I have to stop eating so much!' Whenever you notice this kind of thinking, *the first thing to do is to confront the fear and choose to overeat* by carefully considering the following:

'I don't have to make any changes at all.'
'I'm free to eat anything and everything I can get my hands on.'
'I can continue to eat like this every day for the rest of my life.'

You need to see first that you've got choices before you can make them. Connect to this sense of choice whenever you think about overeating, while you are actually overeating and – *especially* – when you have just finished overeating. When you remember the truth of the free choices that are open to you, you may react in one of these ways:

1　'That's okay with me.' In which case, you continue to overeat.
2　'I don't really feel like I've got much of a choice.' If so, do the written exercises at the end of Chapter 5, reviewing that chapter and Chapter 10.
3　'Yes, but I don't want to continue to live like this.' In which case, identify what it is that you like about eating less, especially those benefits that have nothing to do with the way you look. Then, you make a choice: either to overeat (because you still have the choice to do that!) or to trade the uncomfortable feeling of unsatisfied addictive desire/addictive hunger in order to gain those benefits you want in your life.
4　'Yes, I would eat less, but . . .' Identify any justifications and excuses, and see if you are ready to let go of some of them. Chapters 9 and 10 will help you with this.

Are You Working through Your Addictive Desire?

Many people find it fairly easy to eat less for periods of time because they aren't getting strong feelings of addictive desire. This could be because circumstances in your life just happen not to be triggering it that much. It could also be because you've trained yourself over years to ignore those thoughts whenever you go into your 'being good' phase. After a while, though, it starts to wear thin, and then you can begin to feel as if you're being driven to overeat. You can counteract this by encouraging and facing moments of desire, however subtle they may be, when things are going well. Chapters 6 and 8 will help you with this.

I experience some of my strongest feelings of addictive desire when I am tired. Not because I've thought it out intellectually, but simply because my brain automatically makes the connection that a sugary snack will pick me up fast. I don't have to act on that, though, because I know that would leave me worse off. I know it will be much better for me to get a slower release of glucose and energy from some real food. So (most of the time!) I notice the automatic message from my brain and make the choice I really do want to live with. And I find that a bit of anger at how the food industry has made suckers out of us all for so long really helps me to resist all those packaged 'goodies'.

It will help you to accept that your addictive desire isn't going to go away completely. It will diminish over time, both in intensity and frequency. But when it's there you'll either satisfy it or think yourself through it. When you don't make the deliberate effort to use The Outline to work through the desire (see page 126), your addictive thinking will take over by default.

The default setting of addictive thinking is 'selective memory'. This means you'll remember only the good things about satisfying it and forget the bad consequences – until later on, when you regret what you've done. Your deliberate use of The Outline counteracts this selective memory. The more you use it, the more accessible it becomes.

The real challenge may be in spotting your addictive desire in the first place; Times and Plans make it easier to see. Sometimes a more subtle desire can be difficult to identify and can seem so trivial that you just go ahead and satisfy it without realising. It might be ordering dessert in a restaurant or putting a packet of bagels into your shopping basket. I'm not saying you are not to do these things; just know that when you do it's got nothing to do with nutritional needs and everything to do with addictive desire.

At times it's likely you'll encounter a big cue for your addictive desire. It's likely to produce a stronger urge to overeat, especially if it's a dramatic event such as losing a job or a relationship. Even so, overeating at this time is not inevitable because you still have the option of working through your desire. In time, your addictive desire associated with that kind of situation or emotional state will fade. This is provided you don't reinforce it by satisfying it, and provided you are genuinely choosing to accept it. Like a fire, the desire burns itself out when you stop feeding it. (2)

In Chapter 10 we looked at the primary role of the prefrontal cortex. If you don't make that mental shift to acknowledge choice while you feel addictive desire, you don't engage your prefrontal cortex and you don't make progress.

If you are very keen for the desire to fade, by the way, this signifies that you're not really accepting it. This is an important paradox: the more willing you are to live with unsatisfied desire, the faster it will fade.

It Gets Easier!

At first, all this may seem impossible to sustain, but it gets much easier as new neural pathways are formed. Ways of thinking that were challenging and required a great deal of effort become much more familiar and even automatic because they are now the way your brain works.

Any addictive overeating is in large part automatic and unconscious. This doesn't mean anything about you, that you are hopelessly inadequate in some way. Everything we do in our lives is likely to become automatic. Whether we learn to speak a new language, drive a car or knit a scarf, we struggle with the awkwardness of it at first. We need to be aware of every new nuance, but eventually the skill becomes ours. So don't be too dismayed when you overeat unconsciously and automatically at times. Forgive yourself but know that you can only change things through your awareness, so patiently bring your attention back to the process.

You could think of accepting your addictive desire to eat as the payment you make in order to be in control. Do you prefer to be in control of your overeating? Then this is what it costs. It costs you moments of being aware that you feel uncomfortable and unsatisfied. If you make this payment, control of your addictive overeating is yours to enjoy. If you don't make the payment, you lose it. It's up to you.

The good news is that even if you aren't perfect, you can always make progress. Halfway through a binge, if you can see the value of stopping right there and you choose to work through your desire to continue, that's *something*.

You will go out of control. All you need to do is get up one more time than you fall down. You will make mistakes. All you need to do is notice them and learn from them. That's what failing with style is all about.

This requires courage. You are trying to do something that is extremely important to you, so any amount of failure will cause you to suffer. The 'safe' solution is not to try in the first place or not to try too hard. But then nothing changes.

In the past when I've struggled with this, I've often found it's precisely those times when I've felt the most hopeless that I am closest to a real breakthrough. The solution is right there in the problem, and all it usually takes is one or two very simple things to turn it around. Set yourself a Time, and then make present-time choices either to satisfy and reinforce your addictive desire to eat or to think through these addictive thoughts and feelings in order to gain the benefits you want in your life.

Being in control of my eating means that I feel on top of the world, like there's nothing I can't do. All I need to do is pay the appropriate fee: an uncomfortable feeling of unsatisfied addictive desire. No, it's not easy and it's not magic – *but it works!*

IN OTHER WORDS: DIANA

I had found Gillian's books useful and had started to make changes almost immediately, but it wasn't until I did the course that certain things really hit home and made much more sense.

I decided not to repeat my old patterns of 100 per cent perfection – which was something I had never acknowledged until the course and I have found vital! For me it's completely key. I can have a hiccup in my eating and just forget about it and move on, whereas before I would give up altogether.

I am viewing this as a lifestyle change, reading books on nutrition and self-esteem. I am taking some exercise, not loads, but anything is better than nothing and I want to change my life gradually and not overload by trying to do too much too soon.

At one point the scales came down from the loft and I discovered I had lost a stone. Then I got a little annoyed with myself as it made me start thinking about size and the scales went back into the loft. It took me a ➤

couple of weeks to get my thinking back in the right direction.

When I started to accept how bad sugar is for my health, it was both a revelation and completely terrifying! I was already concerned about diabetes before attending the course, as it runs in my family, and since then I've bought a book on diabetes prevention. It made me realise how close my habits were to slowly killing me. I never knew how eating the wrong things is a death sentence. I could see that clearly regarding smoking, but not eating!

I have the occasional lapse, when I eat too much, but it isn't usually chocolate. I have hardly touched a bar in months and I have had a tub of ice cream in my freezer for over three weeks, which is a record for me! I might eat too much fruit, and I had a lapse with bread the other week. I regularly do that exercise in the supermarket of looking at a pizza and saying, 'I know I can have you, but to be honest to myself, if I buy you I will eat all of you and I like myself too much to do that to my body' – and it works every time! Once I struggled as it was a special offer (buy one, get one free) but I decided not to be seduced by the supermarket superpowers.

Sometimes it's harder when I am with someone else and they egg me on. The other week a friend was pushing for a McDonald's and I got one too, which I quickly justified with 'Well I haven't had any fast food for two months and it will be my 10 per cent slip up'. But whilst eating it I realised I wasn't even enjoying it and left some. But I decline most times and my healthy eating seems to have rubbed off a bit on some of my friends. ➤

> *To be honest I am still slightly overwhelmed at how I*
> *have changed, when I never thought I could.*

Taking Control

- The principle of 'all or none' works on a small scale and is useful to some extent. For example, it could help you to make an 'all or none' choice when you buy a bag of crisps or a packet of biscuits. Be honest about this when you are making your choices. It's *possible* to eat a few, stop and then manage your desire to continue, but it might be easier not to buy it in the first place.

- Set a Time if you don't already have one. 'I'll start again tomorrow' is just another rational and reasonable way to justify addictive eating in the present.

- When was the last time you had a strong addictive desire to eat which you didn't satisfy, even though you could have?

- Feeling some gratitude for your food could be helpful. In our overeating culture we have learned to take food for granted, having little regard for what it is, how it got onto our plate, how it's going to contribute to our wellbeing, and, especially, how fortunate we are to live with this abundance. Consider 'saying grace' before your meal, either privately or with your family. It could be a traditional, religious version or your own creation.

- It's not necessary to make other changes in your life and personality as part of this process. In fact, it's very liberating to establish for yourself that you can take control of your overeating and still be far from perfect – as we all are. Taking control of eating doesn't automatically mean you will become more assertive, popular and clever, nor that you'll get a perfect marriage, exciting sex life or successful career. This may be disappointing – but it takes the pressure off, too!

- Keep this book around you and read it again from time to time, perhaps just dipping in to a few pages or using the Index to find particular topics to review. As you think more about these concepts, and especially when you have used the techniques a bit, coming back to the book will enable you to own it more and make it more meaningful.

Notes

1   Improvements to your health as a result of improved nutrition can take time. Dr Michael Colgan provides some interesting details about this in his book *Optimum Sports Nutrition* (Colgan Institute, 1993): 'The business of nutrition is to build a better body. That has to wait on Nature to turn over body cells. A blood cell lasts 60–120 days. In 3–4 months your whole blood supply is completely replaced. In 6 months almost all the proteins in your body die and are replaced, even the DNA of your genes. In a year all your bones and even the enamel of your teeth is replaced, constructed entirely out of the nutrients that you eat.

'This time course is well illustrated by the course of deficiency diseases. If I remove all the vitamin C from your diet, within 4 weeks blood vitamin C will drop to zero. But you will see no symptoms of disease at 4 weeks. You have to wait until enough of the healthy cells have been replaced by unhealthy cells. It is another 12 weeks before symptoms of scurvy start to ravage your body.

'So when you implement an optimum nutrition program, don't expect rapid results. In one of our studies at the Colgan Institute, runners were supplemented to try to improve their haemoglobin, hematocrit and red blood cell count. But after one month of supplementation, there was no improvement at all. After 6 months, all three indices were significantly increased.'

2   'Pavlov's dogs kept salivating to the bell long after he had stopped giving them the meat. Eventually, however, the bell lost its power to trigger this physiological response . . . The dogs' brains had learned that the bell no longer predicted food.'   *Mind Sculpture* (Bantam, 1999) by Ian Robertson, professor of psychology at Trinity College, Dublin.

Further Help

Gillian Riley is a counsellor and seminar leader who has been helping people to take control of smoking and overeating addictions since 1982. A former smoker and overeater, she brings to her work an understanding of the process of addiction gained through counselling others and through dealing with her own addictive behaviour.

Other books by Gillian Riley are:

How To Stop Smoking And Stay Stopped For Good (Vermilion, 1992) The full version of the smoking programme.

Beating Overeating (Gill & Macmillan/Newleaf, 2001) A pocket-sized, easy-read version of this book.

Quitting Smoking (Gill & Macmillan/Newleaf, 2001) A pocket-sized, easy-read version of *How To Stop Smoking*.

Willpower! (Vermilion, 2003) A good addition to *Eating Less*, expanding on many of the same issues.

Visit www.eatingless.com for information on courses and a CD, as well as useful links.

Index

ALSO AVAILABLE FROM VERMILION
BY GILLIAN RILEY

FREE POST AND PACKING
Overseas customers allow £2.00 per paperback

ORDER:

By phone: **01624 677237**

By post: **Random House Books
c/o Bookpost
PO Box 29
Douglas
Isle of Man IM99 1BQ**

By fax: **01624 670923**

By email: **bookshop@enterprise.net**

Cheques (payable to Bookpost) and credit cards accepted

Prices and availability subject to change without notice.
Allow 28 days for delivery.
When placing your order, please mention if you do not wish to receive
any additional information.

www.randomhouse.co.uk